DISABILITY AND CULTURE: AN INTERNATIONAL AND INTER-PROFESSIONAL PERSPECTIVE

PATRICIA SMITH, PHD
EDITOR

DISABILITY AND CULTURE: AN INTERNATIONAL AND INTER-PROFESSIONAL PERSPECTIVE

PATRICIA SMITH, PHD
EDITOR

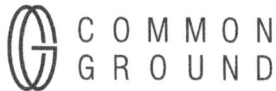

COMMON GROUND

First published in 2015 in Champaign, Illinois, USA
by Common Ground Publishing LLC
as part of the Diversity in Organizations, Communities, & Nations books

Library of Congress Cataloging-in-Publication Data

Disability and culture (Smith)
Disability and culture : an international and inter-professional perspective / [edited by] Patricia Smith.
p. ; cm. -- (Diversity in organizations, communities & nations book series)
Includes bibliographical references.
ISBN 978-1-61229-943-3 (pbk. : alk. paper) -- ISBN 978-1-61229-494-0 (pdf)
1. People with disabilities. 2. People with disabilities--Social conditions. 3. People with disabilities--
Services for. I. Smith, Patricia (Physical therapist), editor. II. Title. III. Series: Diversity in
organizations, communities, and nations (Series)
[DNLM: 1. Cross-Cultural Comparison. 2. Disabled Persons. 3. Community Health Services. 4.
Cultural Competency. 5. Socioeconomic Factors. HV 1568]

HV1568. D553 2014
305.9'08--dc23

2014014947

Cover image photo credit: Phillip Kalantzis-Cope

This book is dedicated to my beloved parents

Iris Victoria Smith
&
Winston George Smith JP

Table of Contents

Acknowledgments

This book is testament of the importance of an understanding of disability and how it is contextualized within cultures. It also reminds us of the need to provide the right kind of physical, attitudinal, socio-political, psychological and mental environment that optimizes the potential of those living with disability.

I therefore firstly give thanks to God, the Supreme Indwelling Intelligence that enables us all to realize our fullest potentials in life and where disability is but an opportunity for this ability to be realized wherever we are in the world.

I would also like to thank all the contributors who, through their involvement in this book have raised the awareness of culture and disability. Thanks for your enthusiasm and responsiveness to comments on your chapters.

Thanks to all my family members and friends. Special thanks to my parents, Winston and Iris Smith who through their love, encouragement and example helped me to realize my goal. Without you both, this would have been an even greater task. Thanks to my brothers and to my sisters Janet Smith & Jacqueline Dawes and to my loving husband Maxwell Garry for your encouragement, and for how you all supported me every step of the way.

Thanks to Professor Keith Gilbert for guiding me and giving me a clear direction. Your input has been invaluable.

Thanks to Common Ground Publishing for your co-operation and patience as the book gradually took form.

Last but by no means least, thanks to all those who read this book and I trust that you will find it a rewarding experience as I have in putting it together.

Dr. Patricia Smith
Editor

About the Authors

Weishe Song was born in China and graduated from Beijing University of Chinese Medicine in 1992 having studied acupuncture, Chinese herbal medicine and Tuina (acupressure) as well as related western medicine subjects. Subsequently he worked for 6 years in the first Hospital of Beijing Medical University in the Faculty of Acupuncture and Herbal Medicine as physician in charge where he conducted a research on cervical spondylosis. Weishe came to the UK in 1998 and now practises acupuncture, Chinese herbal medicine and Tuina in a Chinese medical centre in Kent. From 2000 to 2010, weishe taught Tuina in the London College of Traditional Chinese Medicine. Weishe has been teaching at the University of East London since 2007 where he is the module leader of Acupuncture in Context and TCM Pattern Identification. Weishe is a member of the British Acupuncture Council and the Register of Chinese Herbal Medicine.

Professor Rachael Tribe is a fellow of the British Psychological Society and a Health Professions Council registered psychologist. She has worked and published widely in the areas of migration and mental health, professional and ethical practice in trauma, on interpreters in mental health andhas worked clinically with a range of diverse communities. She is currently based in the School of Psychology at the University of East London. Professor Rachel Tribe has over 30 years of experience of developing clinical services and conducting research both in the UK and abroad.

Dr Fiona McGowan is a senior lecturer in health promotion/ public health at the University of East London. With a nursing and social care background, she later gained her PhD in Medical Sociology at University College London in 2004. Her research focused on the embodiment of masculinity within the context of the life course. More recently, research areas include masculinity, aging and inequality.

Professor John Swain is professor of disability and inclusion at Northumbria University where he has worked as a tutor and researcher for over thirty years. He began his work in the area of disability studies at the Open University and has made numerous contributions to this area.

Sally French works as an associate lecturer with the Open University. She has a professional background in health care and an academic background in the social sciences. Her main interest and work has been in the field of disability studies.

Dr. Patricia Smith is a senior lecturer at the University of East London. She qualified as a physiotherapist and has had several years of clinical practice both in Jamaica and in the UK before developing a career in academia and pursing her doctorate in physiotherapy. Her research interests are community based rehabilitation, cultural competence in higher education curriculum development and qualitative research methodologies. She is actively involved in publishing her current work and developing her research interests.

Professor Threethambal Puckree is executive dean of the Faculty of Health Sciences at the Durban University of Technology in Durban, South Africa. A Fulbright scholar, Professor Puckree earned a PhD in exercise physiology at the State University of New York at Buffalo, a physical therapy license from the University of the State of New York, and a Bachelor of Science in physiotherapy from the University of Durban Westville in Durban. She lectured physiotherapy at the Medical University of Southern Africa in Pretoria and the University of KwaZulu Natal in Durban.

Dr. Keith Gilbert is professor of sports sociology in the School of Health, Sport and Biosciences at the University of East London, United Kingdom.

Dr Otto J. Schantz is a professor of social sciences and dean of the exercise and sport sciences at the University of Koblenz, Germany.

Dr. Melrose Stewart is a lecturer at the University of Birmingham. She holds leads for quality and fitness to practise in physiotherapy within the School of Sport, Exercise and Rehabilitation Sciences. She has recently concluded a 4year term of office as a council member of the Chartered Society of Physiotherapy and was recently elected Vice president. Her PhD focused on the topic of cultural competence in undergraduate physiotherapy education and the topic of equality and diversity continue to be part of the focus of her teaching at undergraduate and postgraduate levels. External to the University, Mel is a member of the judiciary where she sits as a panel member on disability appeals and employment tribunals.

Dr Lesley Dawson, from 1988–1999, headed up the physiotherapy and later occupational therapy programmes at Bethlehem University, in the occupied Palestine territories. On returning to the UK she became programme leader for the accelerated entry level master's programme at University of Brighton, where she was also International Liaison Officer for the School of Health Professions. Since retirement she has been involved in training programmes for therapists in Sub-Saharan Africa with Cerebral Palsy Africa, training tutors in Problem Based Learning at Kathmandu University in Nepal and continuing professional development in various universities in the oPt.

Dr. G Arun Maiya, is associate dean and Professor of Physiotherapy, MCOAHS, Manipal University, Manipal, India

Parul Agarwal is assistant professor of Physiotherapy, MCOAHS, Manipal University, Manipal, India.

Dr. Ronnie Leavitt was an associate professor at the University of Connecticut, USA for 30 years. She has a BS in physical therapy, a Masters in Public Health and a PhD in medical anthropology. Her areas of specialty include cross-cultural competence and international rehabilitation. She is presently retired.

Dr. Aderonke Omobonike Akinpelu is a reader at the University of Ibadan, Nigeria. She obtained her BSc (Physiotherapy) degree in 1977 and PhD (Exercise Physiology) degree in 1990 both from the University of Ibadan. She is an experienced physiotherapy lecturer and her research focus is health outcomes research and Musculoskeletal research. She is currently the acting head of the Department of Physiotherapy, College of Medicine, University of Ibadan.

Mrs. Nse Ayooluwa Odunaiya is a lecturer at the University of Ibadan, Nigeria. She obtained BSc (Physiotherapy) degree in 1991 and M. Ed. (Exercise Physiology) in 1994, both from the University of her Ibadan, Nigeria. She has taught physiotherapy for many years and she is currently running her PhD degree programme in Cardiopulmonary Physiotherapy at the Stellenbosch University, South Africa. Her research focus is epidemiology and prevention of cardiovascular diseases.

Dr. Adesola Christiana Odole is a senior lecturer at the University of Ibadan, Nigeria. She obtained Bachelor of Medical Rehabilitation (physiotherapy) in 1989 from the Obafemi Awolowo University, Ile-Ife, Nigeria, MSc (orthopaedics, sports and recreational physiotherapy) in 2001, PhD degree (orthopaedics, sports and recreational physiotherapy) in 2007 and MSc Biomedical Education in 2011, from the University of Ibadan, Nigeria. She has been teaching physiotherapy since 2008 when she joined the services of the College of Medicine, University of Ibadan in the Department of Physiotherapy. Her research focus is health outcomes research, musculoskeletal research and tele-health.

List of Tables and Figures

Foreword

This book explores the very important issues involving disability and culture, with perspectives and narratives from service users with disability, families living with disability, practitioners, service providers, managers, researchers and academics.

This book pulls together author contributions from experts and practitioners who have a wide ranging and in-depth knowledge and experience, both in the disability movement, and on cultural theories and practices. Their contributions will provide perspectives that challenge old thinking on disability and culture and also provide new material that expands current thinking on the relationship between disability and culture in different contexts. The editor and contributors provide a broad range of personal and inter-professional perspectives on policies and initiatives from around the world that is both authoritative and informative. Contributors argue that culture informs disability and in turn disability informs culture, but more importantly how communities and societies around the world respond to these interactions. The book begins with a historical perspective of disability models and goes on to discuss the cultural context of marginalisation from a socio-political perspective. It then explores the culture of professional practice, including narratives from both patient and carer perspectives; and further explores disability and culture from an international perspective. The book ends by discussing important issues around methodological approaches and cultural considerations in research, and helpfully provides some reflections from each chapter.

All readers should benefit from the information, evidence and narratives in this book, as well as gain inspiration from the experience and enthusiasm of all contributors and the challenges they explore. The interdisciplinary nature of the content particularly enhances the readability of the book and it will appeal to a range of practitioners and academics working in the field of disability and culture, and will also provide a valuable learning resource for a range of health and social care professionals and students, in both pre- and post-graduate study.

Helena C Johnson EdD MEd PgDEdHE BSc Hons MCSP FHEA
Vice-President and Immediate Past Chair of Council. The Chartered Society of Physiotherapy.
Physiotherapy Lead for Strategic Developments, Faculty of Health & Life Sciences, York St John University, UK

Preface

There is no question we live in a mobile world where people travel for new experiences and move home for personal, family, social, political and economic reasons. Our eyes are opened and we are often surprised at the differences in attitudes and beliefs in new environments. Our perceptions of the world as we know it are challenged.

Understanding our own culture and how it has shaped us is imperative to truly understanding ourselves. As health professionals working in a mobile world, understanding cultural differences and similarities is a first step to true cultural competence. As physical therapists, if we want to practice to full potential and deliver services in a truly person centred way we must understand our own culture and we must consider the influence and interaction between culture and disability at individual and community level. The stories and experiences in this book will provide material for reflection and will enrich our professional practice.

Brenda Myers
Secretary General
World Confederation of Physical Therapy (WCPT)

Section I: The Cultural Context of Marginalization: A Socio-political Perspective

Chapter 1: Introduction

Patricia Smith

It was a bright sunny afternoon when I sat on the verandah of my home in Kingston, Jamaica. I often sat at this spot which was shaded by the overhanging branch of a mango tree, when I wanted to think about life. I looked out at the passers-by, some sauntering casually, some walking quickly, but everyone engrossed in their own thoughts and in their own world. I was a teenager at the time; I too was engrossed in my own thoughts, trying to come to terms with my own growing self awareness and trying to make sense of the things that I wanted for my life.

As I looked into the sky, absorbing the warmth of the sunshine, a sudden movement caught the corner of my eye. As I turned to look, I saw her, the same young woman I saw every day passing my gate, dressed in a white tunic and green trousers. This young lady was a physiotherapy student and she shared with me her experience of what physiotherapy was all about. I was moved by the passion with which she spoke and how much it meant to her, especially as there was a severe shortage of physiotherapists in Jamaica. Physiotherapists were in great demand especially in the climate of social and economic changes both globally and nationally in the 1970s. I felt that this was the place where I could make my contribution. I realised my need to become a person who could make a difference to people's lives could be achieved in a helping profession such as physiotherapy. This is what I wanted to do. What was most compelling was that this growing awareness to 'be' and to 'become' such a person, would not be limited to my own ideas of who I am, but would be born out of an interactive relationship with people who lived their lives in different ways. Training as a physiotherapist was more than just a job. In some sense it can be seen as a calling and many years on, my passion for physiotherapy remains. It has brought me to a new part of my life journey, to examine Culture and Disability.

The stories that are told in this book along with the research and literature reviews that has been conducted is about the life experiences of people living with disabilities in different cultures. In some instances it is about the experiences of families coping with a disabled child. These are discussed in the context of the culture of different countries and the experiences of different professionals. It is their story, from their perspective and what living with disability means to them.

It is also about the story of the health professional and their role. It is about community. It's about health care providers. It's about the service users.

The underlying thread throughout this book is the understanding of the 'self', which is consciousness and will (Amen, 2003; Cohen, 1994). In this book it is important, because people living with disability do not exist in a vacuum isolated from others but are interdependent and inter-related with each other and the environment a notion supported by many authors (Amen 2003, Etzioni, 2004, 1998; Arthur, 2000; Farzer, 1999). Community values, norms and cultural practices shape what is known by a person about themselves and their bodies. These are all significant in the context of the country in which people live, their community and their families.

My perspective is one that comes from a combination of experiences that I have had working as a physiotherapist in Jamaica and in the United Kingdom. I endeavour to formulate a conceptual map of my thinking as outlined by Amen (2003) and development as a physiotherapist working in Jamaica. While working in Jamaica in the late 1980s, there were global changes to perspectives of practice in physiotherapy, which began to look at it from a broader perspective (Lolas, 1985; Engel, 1979; Frankenhauser, 1989; Weiss, 1980). On re-locating to the UK in the early nineties, I continued my practice of physiotherapy. I began working as a community (domiciliary) physiotherapist, in a multicultural setting in the UK. My perspective broadened and the challenge to my practice was to understand community physiotherapy from a perspective that related culturally to the people who used the service. This was significant because it made me aware of the need to accept that culture, which may be defined as shared symbols, beliefs and values, is important as a meaning system (Helman, 2001; Kidd, 2002). I came to accept that culture is central to the human experience of illness and disability and as some authors have expressed, is a pre-requisite for understanding all meaningful experiences of man (Burkett, 1991; Benhabib, 2002). The underlying model that was emerging was a problem-solving approach that enabled patients to attain functional independence. As a physiotherapist, I appreciated the need to understand that cultural differences would become increasingly important in carrying out appropriate practice of physiotherapy especially as social mobility has resulted in more people working in cultures other than their own, or in multicultural societies (Noorderhaven, 1999).

This book attempts to address these issues. It attempts to explore and unearth the complex issues surrounding disability and culture. This is done through the insights of colleagues, practitioners, specialists and academics who work in the area of disability and culture. In addition, this book aims to provide the resources for the historical background to the nature of disability from a cultural-global perspective while discussing issues around marginalization and displacement. Lastly, this book looks at challenges and benefits that can be derived from an understanding of the cultural imperatives of disability.

Traditionally, disability has been viewed as impairment or a biological condition arising out of a tragedy or due to a physiological disorder (Barton, 1996). This perspective was largely due to the medical model of disability. However, as perspectives on disability changed, the social model embraced a social viewpoint which later evolved into disability around identity, genetics, eugenics, images and languages. More currently, issues around the environment and its impact on disability has been an area of much debate and over time has taken pre-eminence in the literature (Swain & French, 2008). It is clear that without an enabling environment, whether physical, attitudinal, or behavioural, those living with disability may find it a challenge to perform and function to the best of their ability. Not least, a disabling environment creates dependency and a sense of loss (Swain & French, 2008). Those living with disability have been speaking out to re-balance this imbalance and are pushing to create an environment in which they can experience their full being.

In this book, the arguments are put forward that disability has a wider context than just discussed. How disability is contextualized can be determined from its cultural context. The cultural imperatives that surround disability are vast and wide. The ideas and norms that people in different cultures hold, dictates how they respond to disability and therefore it is hoped that in this text a deeper understanding of the notion of disability and culture will encapsulate the issues. Culture informs disability and disability informs culture and the discussions developed in this book may have important implications on how communities and societies respond to this. It will also promote regeneration and modernization of current practices around disability at all levels of society and provide the means for further research and documentation in the future. This book aims to highlight the common themes that emerge from a national and international perspective on disability and culture.

References

Amen, R (2003) Metu Neter Vol 3. The key to miracles. Khamit Media Trans vision Inc.

Arthur, J (2000) Schools and Community: The Communitarian Agenda in Education. Falmer Press.

Barton, L (1996) *Disability and Society: Emerging Issues and Insights.* Longman Sociology Series.

Cohen, A (1994) *Self Consciousness. An Alternative Anthropology of Identity.* London. Routlege.

Engel, G. L (1979) The Biopsychosocial Model and the Education of Health Professionals. *General Hospital Psychiatry.* 1:156-65.

Etzioni, A (2004) From Empire to Community: A New Approach to International Relations. Palgrave MacMillan

Frankenhaeuser, M (1989) A Biopsychosocial Approach to Work Life Issues. *International Journal of Health Services.* 19:747-58.

Frazer, E (1999) The Problems of communitarian Politics. Unity and Conflict. Oxford Press.

Helman, C. G (2001) *Culture Health and Illness* 4th Edition. Arnold.

Kidd, W (2002) *Culture and Identity: A Skills Based Sociology.*Palgrave.

Kidd, W (2002) *Culture and Identity: A Skills Based Sociology.*Palgrave.

Noorderhaven, N. G. (1999) Intercultural Difference: Consequences for the Physical Therapy Profession.*Physiotherapy*, 85, 504-510.

Swain, J; French, S (2008) Disability on equal terms. Sage Publication Ltd.

Weiss, R. J (1980) The Biopsychosocial Model and Primary Care. *Psychosomatic medicine*, 42, 123-30.

Chapter 2: Disability and Inequalities

Sally French and John Swain

Introduction

Inequality is one of those umbrella terms which seem to encompass all beneath its canopy. Disabled people can indeed face inequality in numerous areas of their lives. Barnes and Mercer (2010) categorized these into three arenas of social life: inequalities in consumption (including income and wealth, access to services, housing, transport and the built environment); production (employment and education); and social interaction (social and political participation, and leisure). In this chapter we focus on two realms. The first is inequalities in life and death. Some people have a better chance of living longer and healthier lives than others. The second is the different social advantages and disadvantages that shape people's lives. Economic inequalities are probably the most often referred to and discussed with the increasing gap between the rich and the poor, individuals and states. Our analysis charts the inextricable linkage between these two realms, with the implication that to confront inequalities in health we need to reduce social inequalities (Graham, 2007).

The chapter then moves on to an examination of the roots of inequality in the dominant paradigm of disability and impairment, particularly as personal tragedy. This can be seen, for instance in the provision of services. Oliver (1990) pointed out that:

> professionals are clearly influenced by cultural images and ideological images of disability as an individual, medical and tragic problem. (p 64)

The inequalities experienced by disabled people are justified from such viewpoints. We also, however, look at the challenges coming from disabled people. These have been generated through the social model of disability which addresses broader socioeconomic issues in analysing inequalities. We concentrate particularly on the affirmative model, a recent derivative of the social model, which confronts the stigmatization of difference and the realisation of positive non-tragic disabled identities.

Disability, Inequalities in Health and Inequalities in Life Chances

To examine the interplay between health and broad social inequalities we need to focus on the many influences on all aspects of health. Dahlgren and Whitehouse (1995) propose a useful model which depicts these influences as layers piled on top of each other.

At the bottom of the pile are biological factors. These include our sex and age and the genes we inherit from our parents. Many diseases become more common as we grow older (for example cancer and cardiovascular disease), some diseases are specific to men or women (for example prostate and ovarian cancer), while others are genetic or congenital in origin (for example cystic fibrosis and haemophilia). Most of these diseases are associated with impairment and disability. Within cultural beliefs poverty can be associated with biological factors. A common line of thought within Western societies is that a person is poor because of personal traits which have caused the person to fail. It is viewed as the individual's personal failure not to climb out of poverty. This thought pattern stems from the idea of meritocracy and its entrenchment within Western thought: those who are worthy are rewarded and those who fail to reap rewards must also lack self-worth.

The second layer focuses on our behaviour. This includes whether or not we smoke cigarettes or eat too much, the amount of exercise we take and how much stress we put ourselves under. Most policy initiatives from government have focused on this layer where attempts have been made to change people's behaviour in order to improve their health (Jones 2000). Wiles (2008), for instance, gives examples of community and Primary Care Trust Partnerships which focus on activities such as walking, cooking, singing, yoga, dancing, craft and improving self esteem. This emphasis on personal behaviour has, however, been criticised. Asthana and Halliday (2006) state that '....the government's strategy suggests an implicit assumption that health inequalities can be reduced without changing overall levels of inequality' (98),There is also a denial of the ways in which the social setting affects our behaviour. Ewles and Simnett (2003) believe that:

> We cannot assume that individual behaviour is the primary cause of ill health.... There is a danger that focusing on the individual detracts attention from the more significant (and, of course, politically sensitive) determinants of health, such as the social and economic factors of racism, relative deprivation, poverty, housing and unemployment. (41)

This emphasis on the individual has implications for disabled people who are expected to accommodate themselves to existing structures in, for instance, employment, education, leisure and housing, although there has been some improvement in recent years as the social model of disability gains influence (Swain, et al 2013). Imrie (2006), talking of housing, states:

> Most dwellings are designed and constructed as 'types' that comprise standard fixtures and fittings that are not sensitive to variations in body form, capabilities and needs..... Builders, building professionals and

others assume that disabled people will be able to adjust to the pre-fixed design of domestic space. (13)

It is notable too that many disabled people would have problems accessing the activities, such as walking, dancing and craft, provided by the Primary Care Trust Partnership mentioned above. Indeed such initiatives tend to be geared to the 'average' person.

The next layer concerns social and community influences. The people around us, including family members, neighbours, colleagues and friends, can influence our health by giving meaning to our lives and providing assistance and support in times of illness, difficulty and stress. Organisations such as the church, leisure clubs and self-help groups may also be important. Conversely these people can have a detrimental effect on our health by neglect, abuse, discrimination or failing to take account of our needs.

The evidence suggests that feelings of isolation are associated with poor physical and mental health. Eberstadt and Satel (2004) note that people who are socially isolated die at twice the rate of those who are well connected and that they are prone to depression which can lead to poor health habits and risk-taking behaviour. Conversely, positive social relations are linked to good health (Asthana and Halliday, 2006, Wiles 2008)As Putman (2000) states:

> As a rule of thumb, if you belong to no groups but decide to join one, you cut your risk of dying in the next year in half. If you smoke but belong to no groups, it's a toss up statistically whether you should stop smoking or start joining. (331)

Assumption about cultural differences with regards to social support can have detrimental effects. For instance discrimination in service provision has been denied and rationalised through myths that Black families prefer "to look after their own". Though the literature documenting the views of black disabled people is sparse, it consistently speaks to experiences of segregation and marginalisation within services. Summarising the evidence from several studies, Butt and Mirza (1996) state:

> The fact that major surveys of the experience of disability persist in hardly mentioning the experience of black disabled people should not deter us from appreciating the messages that emerge from existing work. Racism, sexism and disablism intermingle to amplify the need for supportive social care. However these same factors sometimes mean that black disabled people and their carers get a less than adequate service. (p 94)

Berkman and Melchior (2006) point out that social networks provide opportunities for support, access, social engagement and social and economic advancement allowing individuals to participate in work, community and family life. Social networks can, however, also lead to discrimination, hostility and exclusion.

Disabled people are likely to experience social isolation and discrimination because the barriers within society (environmental, attitudinal and structural) make it difficult or impossible for them to participate as full citizens. This, in turn, is likely to impact adversely on their physical and mental health. Lester and Glasby (2006) point out that mental and physical ill health frequently co-exist. Needing substantial help from relatives and friends can also lead to resentment and breakdown of relationships as the social rule of reciprocity, which underpins most relationships, may be breached. Social isolation and discrimination is likely to be particularly marked for older disabled people who may also experience ageism and may become isolated through retirement, widowhood or the death of friends.

Living and working conditions comprise the next layer of influence. It is well known, for example, that the type of house in which we live and our environment at work can affect our health. Work pressure or noisy neighbours may cause depression and anxiety that can lead to physical ill health (Leon and Walt, 2001) and physical hazards such as dampness, poor architectural design and dangerous work practices can cause disease and injury (Siegnal and Theorell 2006). Living in deprived neighbourhoods also increases the risk of ill health and mortality despite the individual's personal situation (Steptoe, 2006; Wiles, 2008).

It is well known that unemployment is correlated with poor physical and mental health and high mortality rates (Siegnal and Theorell 2006) but employment can also have adverse effects on our health. Low salaried workers have the worst physical and psychosocial environment at work which, in turn, can lead to poor physical and mental health (Dahl et al 2006). Siegnal and Theorell (2006) state that people in jobs where there is high demand and low control are particularly likely to experience stress, although low demand and low control is also stressful particularly if it is linked to low levels of support. High effort and low reward can also lead to ill health because of the lack of reciprocity in the arrangement which is likely to give rise to damaging negative emotions. Certain people, including disabled people, are more likely to accept work of this type through lack of opportunity and choice (Siegnal and Theorell, 2006).

Even disabled people in professional occupations are likely to experience additional stress often because it takes more time and effort to succeed in the job. This is explained by a visually impaired physiotherapist who is talking about the administrative aspects of his job:

> Visually impaired people, with the best computerised systems available, are at a disadvantage because of the amount of time and concentration it takes..... I take time at the end of the day..... I nearly always work my lunch hour. It's got worse over the years. (French 2001:126-7).

Disabled people are also far more likely than non-disabled people to be unemployed (Stanley, 2005) and unemployment is associated with poor physical and mental health (Reine et al, 2004)

Barnes and Roulstone (2005) believe that disabled people should not be judged in terms of whether or not they are involved in paid employment and that the benefits system should be de-stigmatised and more generous to improve their quality of life. It is, for instance, important that they have sufficient resources and access to engage in purposeful activities of their own choosing. Barnes and Roulstone (2005) also believe that the effort involved in coping as a disabled person in a disabling environment should be regarded as work and that their role as employers of personal assistants and the considerable work opportunities for non-disabled people generated by the 'disability industry' should be recognised.

The outermost layer affecting our health concerns are general socioeconomic, cultural and environmental conditions. This includes the economic state of the country, the level of employment, the tax system, the degree of environmental pollution and our attitudes, for example towards ethnic minorities and disabled people. Major research reports over the years have demonstrated that mortality, morbidity and life expectancy are strongly correlated with socioeconomic status with those of the lowest social status being at a considerable disadvantage (Siegrist and Marmot 2006, Power and Kuh 2006, Steptoe 2006).

Lack of an adequate income can impact on health in many ways. Yeandle et al (2008) interviewed men and women on low incomes who reported depression, anxiety, high blood pressure and headaches. They had insufficient fruit and vegetables in their diet and little time for exercise. Women were most affected as they usually put their partners and children first. They also suffered feelings of guilt and failure when they could not give their children what they wanted or what other children enjoyed.

Despite the various influences on our health, the evidence overwhelmingly suggests that broad social factors concerning housing, income, educational level, employment and social integration are more important than our individual behaviour or medical practice and advances (Ewles and Simmett 2003)People of the lowest socio-economic status are at far higher risk, not only of physical illness and early death, but also of accidents, premature births, mental illness and suicide. Most disabled people are of lower socioeconomic status and experience disadvantage over a long period of time. They are, therefore, particularly likely to experience ill health in its broadest sense. Children in the lowest two social classes, for instance, are 16 times more likely to die in fires than children in the highest social class (Sustainable Communities: people, places and prosperity 2005). Smith and Goldblatt (2004) report that of the 66 major causes of death, 62 are more prevalent in the lowest two social classes. It is also the case that men in professional occupations live, on average, seven years longer than men in manual occupations and that the children of manual workers are twice as likely to die before the age of 15 than the children of professionals workers (Naidoo and Wills 2008). In addition Hargreaves (2007) reports that in 2002-2004 Infant mortality was 19% higher among manual workers than professional workers and that the gap had steadily widened.

The Acheson Report (1998), which was based on government commissioned research into inequalities in health, found evidence that every aspect of health is worse for people living in deprived circumstances. Overall this situation has not changed. As Wiles notes'.....across the life span there are inequalities in people's health that follow from their economic position.Poor people are more likely to be in poor health and to die at an earlier age.' (2008:52)

Deprivation and poverty among disabled people is particularly marked in the majority world. This is not just in terms of money but also education, employment, housing, transport, leisure, family life and social relationships

(Barnes and Sheldon 2010). Disabled women and girls are particularly badly affected in all respects. For instance it was estimated by UNESCO in 2007 that only 10% of disabled children in the majority world go to school. Disabled girls and women are particularly badly affected in all respects. In Nepal, for instance, less than 3% of disabled people receive any kind of rehabilitation and 70% receive no education (Dhungama, 2006). The environment is inaccessible in terms of buildings and transport and there is virtually no statutory provision. Dhungama interviewed 30 disabled women and found that 24 experienced humiliation, in the form of taunting and teasing, on the streets. Furthermore one disabled woman who managed to find a job had to leave because there was no accessible toilet. There is a belief in Nepalese society that disabled women bring bad luck to families and 80% remain unmarried even though marriage is the social norm. If married women become disabled they often experience abuse and withdrawal of support from family members and are denied contact with other families leading to isolation. The law in Nepal allows men to divorce their wives if they become disabled.

Kassah (2008) interviewed eight disabled wheelchair users who made their living from begging in Ghana. Kassah explains that disabled people in Ghana receive little education or medical care and even have difficulty finding the resources to feed themselves. Impairment in Ghana is often viewed as a punishment or curse and most disabled people fail to find a marriage partner or may be divorced if they become disabled. Thus for many disabled people begging becomes a means of survival even though it is stigmatised by the government who have tried to eliminate it.

There is substantial evidence, then, that inequalities in health are inextricably interlinked with inequalities in social advantage and disadvantage. It can be argued that this is entirely consistent with the social model of disability. Health inequalities faced by disabled people need to be tackled through broad social change, challenging the discrimination against disabled people and the barriers to full citizenship and social participation.

The Joseph Rowntree Foundation (2008) provides a succinct summary of how poverty and inequality links to cultural ideas:

- Discrimination against people on the grounds of their poverty is a common but relatively unacknowledged feature of life in the UK.
- Such discrimination is sometimes based on views that people living in poverty are inferior or of lesser value. Such attitudes can become embedded as 'povertyism' – a phenomenon akin to racism or sexism
- There are deeply held views amongst the public about the 'deserving' and the 'undeserving' poor in the UK. This is reflected in governments' resistance to highlighting wealth redistribution as a means of combating poverty.[1]

Similar statements can be made about cultural ideas relating to disability and thus discrimination faced by disabled people in poverty is compounded.

---

[1]www.jrf.org.uk/publications/poverty-uk-denial-peoples-human

Personal Tragedy, Non-tragedy, and Service Provision

Where, then, are the foundations of inequality? A major basis is the tragedy view, or model, of disability and impairment. This model is integral to other individual models of disability. The tragedy model portrays disability as a biological condition and a limitation (Saxton, 2000), 'as a deficit, a personal burden and a tragedy' (Wilder, 2006:2), as an enemy (Mason, 2000), as 'abject and abhorrent' (Darke, 2004:103), and as '"abnormal" and something to be avoided at all costs.' (Oliver and Barnes, 1996:66). Disabled people are perceived as being robbed of any enjoyment in life and as a burden to society (Saxton, 2000).Parens and Asch state:

> There are many widely accepted beliefs about what life with disability is like for children and their families......They include assumptions that people with disabilities lead lives of relentless agony and frustration and that most marriages break up under the strain of having a child with a disability (2000:20).

It is clear that there are aspects of people's behaviour and attitudes, other than viewing disabled people as tragic, which may lead to unequal treatment. For instance, the needs or indeed rights of disabled people frequently involve non-disabled people in learning new skills (sign language, for instance) or putting themselves out in various ways, such as giving more time or adjusting the way they normally do things. Nevertheless, despite some variation, the tragedy view of disability is widespread across cultures (Coleridge, 1993; Ingstad and Reynolds Whyte, 1995; Barnes and Mercer, 2005) and throughout history (Stiker, 1997; Longmore and Umanski, 2001; Borsay, 2005) and remains so entrenched in society today it has become an ideology. Oliver explains that:

> .....ideologies are so deeply embedded in social consciousness generally that they become 'facts'; they are naturalised. Thus everyone knows that disability is a personal tragedy for individuals so 'affected'; hence ideology becomes common sense (1993:50).

This model is rooted in everyday language. The words used to describe disabled people are invariably negative or passive. Many words in common use, for example 'short-sighted', meaning lack of insight, show how deeply ingrained negative perceptions of disability are. The very words 'disabled' (not able) and 'invalid' (not valid) indicate the lowly status disabled people have within society.

The denigration and misrepresentation of disabled people in language is widespread across the world. For instance, in Chinese the character for 'blind' comprises the characters for eye and drum thus depicting blind people as musicians, and the character for physical deformity depicts a worm (Stone, 1999).

Descriptions of disabled people frequently have tragic overtones, for example 'sufferers' and 'victims' and disabled people are often spoken of as an homogeneous group, for example 'the disabled' and 'the deaf' which is reflected in the titles of many leading charities such as Riding for the Disabled. Disabled people are repeatedly labelled by their impairments ('he's a paraplegic', 'she's an amputee') as if the 'tragedy' of impairment renders everything else about them irrelevant and which gives them a way of being and an identity. This language also stereotypes disabled people rather than regarding them as unique individuals.

It is also true that labels ascribed to disabled people sometimes appear, on the surface, to be very positive. For instance, disabled people may be described as cheerful, clever and courageous: indeed, it is not unusual for disabled people to be regarded as courageous simply for living with an impairment, thus underlining the supposed tragedy of impairment.

The tragedy model has underpinned a great deal of oppressive policy and practice towards disabled people. With the tragedy model in place, there has been little motivation to adjust the environment to take the needs of disabled people into account. The response instead has been to separate disabled people from society and incarcerate them in institutions such as hospitals and residential schools. The tragedy model underpins ostensible treatment and rehabilitation. For instance, the continuing perceived imperative for the prevention of impairment using prenatal screening and abortion and the development of genetic technologies for the eradication or 'cure' of impairments devalues disabled people and their lives.

A central tenet of the tragedy model is that disabled people should strive to be 'normal' and 'independent', whatever the cost to themselves, in order to reduce the 'tragedy' that has befallen both them and their families (French, 1994). Deaf children, for example, were prevented from using sign language and were punished for using it (Humphries and Gordon, 1992; Dimmock, 1993; Corker, 1996). Lapper, who was born with no arms and short legs recalls the obsession with 'normality' at the residential home and school she attended:

> The staff were very keen that we all became proficient in the use of our artificial limbs. The add-on limbs were considered a fundamental aspect of our being able to function properly and fulfil the ultimate aim of the home.....they had great faith in those artificial limbs and thought that if we would only practice and use them regularly we would soon be picking up even the most delicate items without breaking or damaging them. But we all instinctively knew those sorry bits of metal were never going to fulfil their hoped-for potential (2005: 35).

If disabled people resist these pressures to be 'normal' they often meet with anger and resistance. Sutherland states:

> I've known a few people who, as adults, have refused to walk even though they could because it's just not worth the effort. And people have got angry with them, often. They've been labelled lazy and all sorts of things. They're definitely considered odd if they choose to be in a wheelchair, in the same way that you're considered odd if you don't struggle to do something that you can actually do even though it takes you six hours (1981:69).

The dominant personal tragedy view of disability has been challenged in many ways by disabled people, including through disability arts. Swain and French (2000) drew on the documented views of disabled people to propose the affirmative model of disability and impairment. It is an extension of the social model. Whereas the social model grew in opposition to the medical model, the affirmative model grew, they claim, in opposition to the tragedy model. It is a non-tragedy view of disability and impairment. The affirmative model is developing out of the individual and collective experiences of disabled people that directly confront the personal tragedy model not only of disability but also of impairment. The emergence of the affirmative model is associated with the growth of the disability arts movement. Many pieces of art by disabled people, including poems, stories and visual art, can be seen as political statements celebrating difference.

From the documented views of disabled people, far from being tragic, being disabled and impaired can have benefits for lifestyle, and can be a source of pride. To give just one example, for Tom, impaired through the drug thalidomide, being disabled provided a context in which he created opportunities and choices:

> Life is very good.....being born with no arms has opened up so many different things that I would never have done. My motto is 'in life try everything'. I wouldn't have that philosophy if I'd been born with arms. (BBC Radio 4Broadcast 2002)

Swain and French (2008) identified a number of features by which this model is characterised. It is about:

- Being different and thinking differently about being different, both individually and collectively,
- The affirmation of unique ways of being situated within society,
- Disabled people challenging presumptions about themselves and their lives in terms of how they differ from what is thought to be average or the norm,
- The assertion on disabled people's own terms of human embodiment, lifestyles, quality of life and identity,
- Ways of being that embrace difference.

This way of thinking directly confronts the personal tragedy model not only of disability but also of impairment, which is the central focus of the tragedy model. Indeed, disability is seen as being caused by impairment and often confused with impairment. From his research into this model Cameron (2008) came to a new definition of impairment which dissociates it from functional ability and the medical model:

> Physical, sensory, emotional and cognitive difference, divergent from culturally valued norms of embodiment, to be expected and respected on its own terms in a diverse society.

From the documented viewpoint of disabled people, far from being tragic, being disabled can have benefits.

In challenging the presumptions of tragedy built into and perpetuated by professional intervention, a non-tragedy view addresses unequal power relations including those that reverberate throughout professional and service systems. To engage with this we shall look toward a research project which examined Centres for Independent Living (CILs) and the work of disabled people as service providers (Barnes and Mercer, 2006). CILs are a particular type of self-help organization, exclusively run and controlled by disabled people themselves. They provide a new and innovative range of services and support systems designed to enable people with impairments to adopt a lifestyle of their own choosing, in contrast to other professionally dominated provision that have focused almost exclusively on medical treatments and therapies within institutional settings. Decision making and working practices within CILs are controlled by disabled people who do not regard disability as an individualized tragedy but as a civil rights issue. Their work is geared towards the fulfilment of disabled people's needs on their own terms and viewing disabled people as active, capable citizens who are restricted, not by impairment, but by a disabling society.

Derbyshire CIL set out and worked towards meeting seven needs, seen as putting the social model into action:

- information
- counselling
- housing
- technical aids
- personal assistance
- transport
- access

Two main themes emerged in the research conducted by Barnes and Mercer (2006): choice and control; and peer support. In relation to a non tragedy approach the CILs have a number of implications:

- Their work speaks directly to disabled people's choice and control over services and intervention, grounded in user-led organisations.
- They speak too to the non-disabled/disabled social divide. The non-tragedy model is founded in experiences of impairment and disability and the self-empowerment to confront presumptions of tragedy.
- The work of the CILs also gives expression and translates into action the collective and shared experiences of non-tragedy. The tragedy view is quintessentially individual.

The affirmative model confronts the role, function and purpose of professionals in providing services. Ballantyne and Muir (2008) discuss the implications of an affirmative model for changing policy, provision and practice within occupational therapy. They state that:

> The affirmative model will, by implication, challenge therapists to redefine their concept of the service users. A redefinition of service users, acknowledging positive elements of their experience of impairment and disability and locating them within a social context, will lead therapists to refocus their service provision. (p 146)

Conclusion

It can be seen from this account that issues of inequality and disability are both fundamental and complex. We have, however, only touched the surface given that disabled people can encounter inequality through multiple oppression, being from an ethnic minority community, being young or old, or gay or lesbian. In the face of different forms of discrimination and multiple discrimination, as well as the vested interests that obstruct change, there can be no simple solution to overcoming health and broad social inequalities. Inequalities seem solidified in dominant cultural beliefs in the personal tragedy of disability and equality. Successful change will only result from collective commitment and action and it is essential that the 'voice' of disabled people, both individual and collective, directs any change that is made.

References

Acheson, D. (1998) *Independent Inquiry Into Inequalities in Health*, London, The Stationery Office.

Asthana, S. and Halliday J. (2006) *What Works in Tackling Health Inequalities?*, Bristol, Polity Press.

Ballantyne, E. and Muir, A., 2008. In practice from the viewpoint of an occupational therapist. In: J. Swain and S. French, ed. *Disability on equal terms*. London: Sage.

Barnes, C. and Mercer, G., 2006. *Independent futures: creating used-led disability services in a disabling society*. Bristol: Policy Press.

Barnes, C. and Mercer, G., 2010. *Exploring disability: a sociological introduction*. 3rd ed. Cambridge: Polity Press.

Barnes, C. and Sheldon A. (2010) Disability Politics and Poverty in a Majority World Context, *Disability and Society*, 25, 7, p771-782.

Barnes, C. and Roulstone A. (2005) 'Work' is a four-letter word: disability, work and welfare, In Roulstone A. and Barnes C. (eds.), *Working Futures? Disabled People, Policy and Social Inclusion*, Bristol, Policy Press.

BBC Radio 4 Broadcast (2002, June) *Thalidomide:40 Years On*.

Berkman, L. F. and Melchior M. (2006) The Shape of Things to Come: how social policy impacts social integration and family structure to produce population health, In Siegrist J. And Marmot M. (eds.) *Social Inequalities in Health: new evidence and policy implications*, Oxford, Oxford University Press.

Borsay, A. (2005) *Disability and Social Policy in Britain since 1750: a history of exclusion*. Basingstoke: Palgrave Macmillan.

Butt, J. and Mirza, K. (1996) *Social Care and Black Communities*, London: Race Equality Unit.

Cameron, C., 2008. Further towards an affirmative model. In: T. Campbell, ed. *Disability studies: emerging insights and perspectives*. Leeds: The Disability Press.

Coleridge, P. (1993) *Disability, Liberation and Development*. Oxford: Oxfam.

Corker, M., (1996) *Deaf Transitions: Images and Origins of Deaf Families, Deaf Communities and Deaf Identities*. London: Jessica Kingsley.

Dahl, E, Fritzell J., Lahelma E.(2006) Welfare State Regimes and Health Inequalities, In Siegrist J. And Marmot M. (eds.) *Social Inequalities in Health: new evidence and policy implications*, Oxford, Oxford University Press.

Dahlgren, G. and Whitehouse M. (1995) *Policies and Strategies to Promote Social Equity in Health,* Stockholm, Institute for Futures Studies.

Darke, P. (2004) The changing face of representation of disability in the media, in J. Swain, S. French, C. Barnes and C. Thomas (eds.) *Disabling Barriers – Enabling Environments*, 2nd edn. Sage: London.

Dhungama, B. M. (2006) The Lives of Disabled Women in Nepal: Vulnerability without support, *Disability and Society*, 21, 2, p133-146.

Dimmock, A. F. (1993) *Cruel Legacy: an introduction to the record of deaf people in history*. Edinburgh: Scottish Workshop Publications.

Eberstadt, N. and Satel, S. (2004) *Health and the Income Inequality Hypothesis*, Washington, The AEI Press.

Ewles, L. and Simnett I. (2003) *Promoting Health: A practical guide,* (5th ed.), London, Bailliere Tindall.

French, S. (1994) 'The disabled role', in S. French (ed.) *On Equal Terms: working with diabled people.* Oxford: Butterworth-Heinemann.

French, S. (2001) *Disabled People and Employment: a study of the working lives of visually impaired physiotherapists*, Aldershot, Ashgate.

Graham, H., 2007. *Unequal lives: health and socioeconomic inequalities*. Maidenhead: Open University Press.

Hargreaves S. (2007) Gaps between UK Social Groups in Infant Mortality are Widening, *British Medical Journal*, 384, 7589, p335.

Humphries, S. and Gordon, P. (1992) *Out of Sight: the experience of disability 1900-1950*, Plymouth: Northcote House Publishers.

Imrie, R. (2006) *Accessible Housing: quality, disability and design*, Abingdon, Routledge.

Ingstad, B. and Reynolds Whyte, S. (eds.) (1995) *Disability and Culture*. Los Angeles: University of California. .

Jones,L. (2000) Behavioural and Environmental Influences on Health, In Katz J., Peberdy A., and Douglas J. (eds.) *Promoting Health: Knowledge and Practice.* (2nd ed.), Basingstoke, Palgrave.

Joseph, Rowntree Foundation (2008) www.jrf.org.uk/publications/poverty-uk-denial-peoples-human

Kassah, A. K. (2008) Begging As Work: A study of people with mobility disabilities in Accra Ghana, *Disability and Society*, 23, 2, p163-170.

Lapper, A. (2005) *My Life in My Hands*. London: Simon and Schuster.

Leon, D. and Walt G. (2001) Poverty, Inequality and Health in International Perspective: a divided world? In Leon D. and Walt G. (eds.), *Poverty, Inequality and health: an international perspective,* Oxford, Oxford University Press.

Lester, H. and Glasby, J. (2006) *Mental Health Policy and Practice*, Houndmills, Palgrave Macmillan.

Longmore, P. K. and Umansky, L. (eds.) (2001) *The New Disability History*. New York: New York University Press.

Mason, M. (2000) Incurably Human. London: Working Press.

Naidoo, J. and Wills, J. (2008) *Foundations of Health Promotion*. Oxford: Elsevier.

Oliver, M. (1990) *The Politics of Disablement*. Basingstoke: Macmillan.

Oliver, M. (1993) 'Disability: a creation of industrialised societies?' in J. Swain, V. Finkelstein, S. French and M. Oliver (eds.) *Disabling Barriers: Enabling Environments*. Buckingham: Open University Press.

Oliver, M. and Barnes, C. (1996) *Disabled People and Social Policy: from exclusion to inclusion*. London: Longman.

Parens, E. and Asch, A. (eds.) (2000) *Prenatal Testing and Disability Rights*. Washington DC: Georgetown University Press.

Power, C. and Kuh, D. (2006) Life Course Development of Unequal Health, In Siegrist J. And Marmot M. (eds.) *Social Inequalities in Health: new evidence and policy implications*, Oxford, Oxford University Press.

Putman, R. D. (2000) *Bowling Alone: the collapse and revival of American community*, New York, Simon and Schuster.

Reine I., Novo, M. and Hammarstrom, A (2004) Does the Association Between Ill Health and Unemployment Differ Between Young People and Adults: results from a 14 year follow up study with a focus on psychological health and smoking, *Public Health*, 118, 5, 337-345.

Saxton, M. (2000) Why members of the disability community oppose prenatal diagnosis and selective abortion, in E. Parens and A. Asch (eds.) *Prenatal Testing and Disability Rights*. Washington: Georgetown University Press.

Siegnal, J. and Theorell, T. (2006) Socio-economic Position and Health: the role of work and employment, In Siegrist J. and Marmot M. (eds.) *Social Inequalities in Health: new evidence and policy implications*, Oxford, Oxford University Press.

Siegrist, J. and Marmot, M (2006) Social Inequalities in Health: basic facts, In Siegrist J. And Marmot M. (eds.), *Social Inequalities in Health: new evidence and policy implications*, Oxford, Oxford University Press.

Smith, B. and Goldblatt, D. (2004) Whose Health Is It Anyway? In Hitchliffe S. and Woodward K. (eds.), *The Natural and the Social: uncertainty, risk, change* (2nd ed.), London, Routledge.

Stanley, K. (2005) The Missing Million: the challenges of employing more disabled people, In Roulstone A. and Barnes C. (eds.), *Working Futures: disabled people, policy and social inclusion*, Bristol, Policy Press.

Steptoe, A. (2006) Psychological Processes Linking Socio-economic Position with Health, In Siegrist J. And Marmot M. (eds.), *Social Inequalities in Health: new evidence and policy implications*, Oxford, Oxford University Press.

Stiker, H. (1997) *A History of Disability*. Ann Arbor: University of Michigan Press. *Sustainable Communities: people, places and prosperity. A five year plan from the office of the deputy prime minister* (2005), London, The Stationery Office.

Sutherland, A. T. (1981) *Disabled We Stand*. London: Souvenir Press.

Swain, J. and French, S. (2000) 'Towards an affirmation model of disability', *Disability& Society*, 15(4): 569-582.

Swain, J. and French, S. 2008. Affirming identity. In: J. Swain and S. French, ed. *Disability on equal terms*. London: Sage.

Swain, J. French, S. Barnes C. and Thomas, C. (eds.) (2013) Disabling Barriers – Enabling Environments, 3rd edn. London: Sage.

UNESCO (2007) EFA Global Monitoring Report 2007 - Strong Foundation: Early Childhood Care and Education, Paris, United Nations Educational, Scientific and Cultural Organisation.

Wilder, E. (2006) *Wheeling and Dealing: Living with Spinal Cord Injury*. Nashville: Wanderbilt University Press.

Wiles, F. (2008) Diverse Communities and Resources for Care, Open University course K101 *Understanding Health and Social Care*, Block 3, Milton Keynes, Open University.

Yeandle, S., Escott K., Grant L. and Batty E. (2008) Women and Men talking about Poverty. In Johnson J. and De Souza C. (eds.), *Understanding Health and social Care: an introductory reader* (2nd ed.), London, Sage.

Chapter3: Paralympic Sport, Marginalization and the Media[2]

Keith Gilbert& Otto J. Schantz

Introduction

Mass media plays an important role in all societies and according to a broadly shared view by experts in mass communication they have the potential to influence, to control and to innovate, and within the disability context they offer "a major source of definitions and images of social reality"; indeed, they provide "the primary key to fame and celebrity", and impart a"source of an ordered and public meaning system which provides a benchmark for what is normal, empirical and evaluative" (McQuail, 1993, p.1). These aspects are of great relevance in the field of sports which is often characterized by the athletes struggle for fame and celebrity and where the normal criteria are to disregard people with disabilities. In many ways the problems encountered by individuals with a disability also impact on the Paralympic athlete.

The way mass media cover Paralympic sports still seems to be characterized by two extremes: either they do glamorous hagiography by transforming the athletes into tragic heroes who have overcome their terrible fate or they just ignore disability sports and reduce the Paralympic athletes into the "zeros" category. In completing this chapter we feel that thefollowing critical analysis of the media discourse and presentation could indeed contribute to lasting change.

Media Effects

The Media construct almost all of our knowledge beyond direct experience and they play a key role in shaping our representations of the world (cf. Früh, 1994;

---

[2]Original sections of this chapter were first produced for the book by Otto Schantz and Keith Gilbert (2012) titled 'Heroes or Zeroes: The media's perceptions of Paralympic sport', Common-ground Publishing, Illinois. U. S. A. We thank the publisher for allowing us to reproduce sections here.

Luhmann, 1996; McCombs, 1994)[3]. Their influence on our daily lives is so pervasive that often our thoughts, behaviors, styles and opinions are based on the mass media's actual construction of knowledge (Kellner, 1995, pp. 151-152). Early studies of the media effects on society have claimed that one of the major influences of the mass media is to reinforce existing norms and attitudes (Lazarsfeld & Merton, 1948). Even though it is uncertain if and in how far the media discourse reflects and influences the opinions and attitudes of the public (Schönbach, 1992) some research indicates, that under certain conditions the media might serve to change public opinion (Berelson, 1960; Kellner, 1995; Noelle-Neumann, 1994). Transactional theories regarding media impact indicate the interdependence between news selection/construction by the media and consumers' attention. Indeed, there is also substantial research stating that the family's and peer group's influence is more pertinent than the media's, but mass media have the power to inform or not to inform about an event or to construct reality from a particular perspective (Berghaus, 1999). They thus have power to influence our perspectives of the so-called "disabled sports" and in particular the Paralympic Games. In this regard the agenda-setting approach of mass media (Dearing & Rogers, 1996; Erbring et al., 1980) suggests that media continually create subject matter which interests and influences people to talk about and discuss issues further. In fact, different studies indicate, that the public's knowledge about and attitudes towards individuals with disabilities are mostly constructed indirectly, often by the mass media (Hackforth, 1988; Stautner, 1989; Farnall & Smith, 1999). This is significant because news and entertainment media seem to have played a significant role on the manner in which society stereotypes people with a disability (Farnall & Smith, 1999; Greenberg & Brand, 1994; Oakes et al., 1994).

Although, the most influential mass medium is television, the print media appears to offer marginal sports, sports for all and sport for people with disabilities a chance to become better known by the public, while TV coverage focuses mainly on show and spectacle (Hackforth, 1994). However, even sport spectators who watch television still seem to consult newspapers regularly in order to get further information about sport (Oehmichen, 1991). This is interesting in particular for information regarding athletes and some other groups who are marginalized within society.

Marginalization of Athletes with a Disability

Over the past twenty years the media coverage of sport has undergone a process of spectacularization and sport has gradually become a commodity; whose media value is "determined by the size and composition of audience and how it can deliver to potential advertisers and sponsors"(Maguire, 1993, pp. 38-39). However, generally the whole range of media doesn't seem to have a great

---

[3] Jean Baudrillard (1991) takes an extreme position and completely separates the real events and the reality constructed by the media. Paraphrasing the title of a novel from Jean Giraudoux he states in a provocative way: "La guerre du Golfe n'a pas eu lieu" - (The Gulf War never happened).

opinion regarding the value of sport for persons with disabilities. Indeed, sport media coverage still marginalizes the Paralympic athletes as they do not meet the socially constructed ideals of physicality, masculinity and sexuality which according to Karin DePauw represent three key aspects of sport (DePauw, 1997). This concept defines physicality as the "socially accepted view of able bodied physical ability" (DePauw, 1997p. 421), masculinity includes "aggression, independence, strength, courage" and sexuality is defined as the "socially expected and accepted view of sexual behavior" (DePauw, 1997p. 421). Concerning the key aspects sexuality and physicality it is widely believed that, even more than the sexual behavior or the physical ability, appearance in form of stereotyped erotic attractiveness of the sporting body, especially the female body, plays an important role in the media coverage of sports (Bette, 1999; Guttmann, 1996; Pfister, 1989; Rowe, 1999). A striking example is beach volleyball where the sexual attractiveness is emphasized by specific official rules and regulations limiting the covered surface of the female body. It could be argued therefore that, female athletes with a disability are exposed to a form of 'threefold discrimination', as in general they do not fit the social constructs of able-bodied athletes, including those of masculinity and sexual attractiveness. Recently Dame Tanni Gray Thompson, the ex British Paralympian, was being interviewed on the BBC television programme 'Hard Talk' but mid interview the program was unceremoniously cut and the BBC switched to the boring live trial of ex Egyptian president Mubarack. The BBC was thus forced to show a topical event [like all the other channels] but in doing so not only succeeded in marginalizing the Dame but also in promoting the concept that coverage of disability is worthless. If this occurs to the top level members of society then we can only imagine what the television producers think of disabled athletes and disabled individuals in local communities.

Sport Specific Newsworthiness

We can draw conclusions about the consumers' attentions and attitudes towards the Paralympics and the athletes with disabilities by analyzing how the print media construct the reality of these Games or disabled athletes in order to interest the recipients. This can be achieved principally by examining information that media consider to be newsworthy.

According to the theoretical concept of news factors (Bell, 1991; Eilders, 1997; Galtung & Ruge, 1965), sport specific coverage of the Paralympic sport should focus on similar topics, which are considered to be newsworthy on the usual sports pages. When representing sports, the mass media in general emphasize action, records, elite performances, aggressive behavior, heroic actions, drama, emotions and celebrities (sport stars). However, the newspapers also focus on performances, results, statistics, and behind the scene stories. Photos capture celebrities, actions and emotions (Becker, 1983; Coakely, 1994; Hackfort, 1988; Krüger, 1993). Along with this, newspaper sport reporting emphasises a number of important general news values, for example the frequency criterion as a continuing activity, or simplicity due to the nature of winning or losing. Sports then are "consonant with expectations, their script follows a familiar pattern" (Bell, 1991, 160) and at the same time the unexpected outcome creates excitement (Elias & Dunning, 1970).

Another inherent condition of sport coverage involves play and competition between nations, which allows the newsworthy reporting of ethnocentric issues. Sport personalities are depicted as celebrities and as such are often cast to the forefront of public interest. Sport is organized conflict with losers and winners all of which can be highlighted in the press. Negativity, which is another important news value, can thus be represented by "bad guys" who take drugs or individuals who abuse the referee (Becker, 1983; Bell, 1991; Hackfort 1988; Krueger, 1993).

Reporting Disability in the Print Media

Studies in the 1990s indicated that the quality and quantity of print media coverage of people with disabilities were of a low standard and the media often portrayed these people unrealistically and stereotypically (Keller et al., 1990; Lachal, 1990a; 1990b; Nelson, 1994; Shapiro, 1993; Yoshida et al., 1990). Riley II (2005, p. ix), the co-founder of WeMedia, the first multimedia company devoted to people with disabilities, ascertains that we still can find a "patronizing, trivializing, and marginalizing ur-narrative of disability in the media today". Recently, in his qualitative and quantitative analysis of German newspapers, Scholz found that these papers still use a cliché-ridden style, focus on medical perspectives or mention disabilities even if they add no information of interest to the reported topics (Scholz, 2010). Longmore (1985) explained these stereotypical media portrayals as a reflection of the public's fears and anxieties. He stated, "We harbor unspoken anxieties about the possibilities of disablement, to us or to someone close to us. What we fear we often stigmatize and shun and sometimes seek to destroy" (Longmore, 1985 p. 32).

As early as 1985 Zola (p.8) observed that in films people with disabilities were most often portrayed as victims, relatively seldom as heroes or villains, and two of the most metaphorical traits that can be found are the marriage between media and disability sports coverage (Hall, 1997). Nelson (1994) listed seven major stereotypes as they were shown in the American media: the person with disabilities as "pitiable and pathetic" (p. 5), as "supercrip" (p. 6), as "sinister, evil, and criminal" (p. 6), as "better-off dead" (p. 7), as "maladjusted" (p. 8), as "burden" (p. 8), and as "unable to live a successful life" (p 9). From a semiological perspective Woodill (1994) distinguished different types of metaphors of disabilities in popular cultures, including newspaper presentations: The humanitarian ("disability as misfortune"), the medical ("disability as sickness"), the outsider ("disabled person as other"), the religious ("disability as divine plan"), the retribution ("disability as punishment"), the social control ("disability as threat"), and the zoological metaphor ("disability person as pet, disability as entertainment"), (Woodill, 1994 p. 209). Of interest is the fact that Clogston (1994) divided newspaper coverage of people with disabilities into two distinct types: the traditional and the progressive models. The traditional model "views persons with disabilities as dysfunctions in a medical or economic way" (p. 46) and as such they must be cared for medically or economically by society. Another attitude of the traditional perspective is to regard them as "super crips" for the way they master their fates (Sandfort, 1982; Clogston, 1994, Shapiro,

1993; Zola, 1985; Hardin & Hardin, 2004, Silva & Howe, 2012). The progressive model views "the major limiting aspect of a person's disability as lying in society's inability to adapt its physical, social, or occupational environment as well as its attitudes, to accept those who are physically different" (Clogston, 1994, 47). A progressive coverage of people with disability would consider individuals as different, accepting their otherness as part of a cultural pluralism and thereby applying a pluralistic rationality (Lyotard, 1983, 13), whereas the traditional discourse considers individuals with a disability as different and inferior to the hegemonic mainstream, thus exerting an excluding rationality (Foucault, 1961).

Coverage of Sport for Individuals with Disabilities in the Media

Studies about media coverage of sport activities of people with disabilities are still relatively rare but there seems to be a growing interest for this topic (Génolini, 1995; Kauer & Bös, 1998; Schantz & Marty, 1995; Schantz & Gilbert 2001, Schantz & Gilbert, 2008). Schimanski (1994) conducted one of the most important studies. When comparing German and North American journals for the period from 1984 to 1992 he found an increasing coverage of sport for persons with disabilities and observed that this coverage moved progressively from other headings to the sports pages. These findings were partly confirmed by the results of Schantz and Marty (1995) who analyzed the French daily sports journal *L'Équipe* and observed increasing frequencies of articles about sport for people with disabilities during a seven-year period from 1987 to 1993. But this evolution did not really improve the rather marginal role of sports for individuals with disabilities in this newspaper. The authors also observed that the articles often showed pity[4] for the athletes or focused on the way the people were coping with their fate instead of referring to the athletes and their performances in a sport specific manner.Paralympic athletes, as we know, would prefer to be reported for their physical feats and not their disability (Schantz & Alberto 1999).

Génolini (1995) analyzed newspaper clippings concerning physical activities for people with intellectual disabilities collected by French sports associations from 1979 to 1986. He found that these persons were portrayed as "gentle monsters" (Génolini, 1995 p. 60), an image that is in-between the beast (mythical aspect) and the child (aspect of educability). The medical model still seems to dominate media coverage. Journalists contribute to perpetuate the biomedical model of disability as they often use medical terminology to describe and to locate the disabilities of athletes (Smith & Thomas 2005; Thomas & Smith, 2003; Howe, 2008; Schell & Duncan, 1999; DePauw, 2000).

---

[4] Persons with disabilities need respect recognition and rights: Pity may be a first step for individuals and later lead to a form of regression if recognition, respect, and rights are lacking. Indeed, "Not its weakness, but its limits make pity questionable; pity is never enough" (Nicht die Weichheit, sondern das Beschränkende am Mitleid macht es fragwürdig, es ist immer zu wenig" Horkheimer, Adorno 1989 [1947] p. 121). Cf. Also Gill (1994), a disability activist, who asks for recognition and respect of difference.

Sport Coverage and Discrimination Based on Severity of Disability

The print media coverage of sport for individuals with disabilities appears to privilege some specific types of disabilities: The main group of individuals with a physical disability, which was by far the most over-represented, is the wheelchair fraternity (Schantz & Marty, 1995; Schimanski, 1994). This is perhaps because the public's perception of the athlete with disabilities is historically that of individuals in wheelchairs. Lachal (1990a; 1990b) who analyzed regional French newspapers from 1977 and 1988 found that in 1988 about half (49%) of the articles about disabilities concerned physical (motor) disabilities, 29% disability in general, 11.5 % sensorial disabilities, 7% intellectual deficiencies, and 3.5% "other" disabilities (Lachal, 1990a, p. 39). Topics concerning athletes with a mental disability figured rarely in the French *L'Équipe*, studied by Schantz & Marty (1995). In their content analysis of TV coverage of the Atlanta Games, Schell and Duncan (1999, p. 44) found that CBS featured less visible, war induced, or acquired disabilities more likely than others.

Sport Coverage and Discrimination Based on Gender and Race

Gender bias reporting in the media is another important area which requires further research in the Paralympic arena. Although in the able-bodied print media there have been relatively great numbers of researchers who have focused on gender biased media coverage (Duncan et al., 1991; Duncan, 1990; Eastmann & Billings 2000; Haller, 2000; Hardin & Hardin, 2005; Hardin, 2003; Jones et al., 1999; Pappous et al., 2011; Smart, 2001; Urquhart & Crossmann, 1999; Wann et al., 1998). In an analysis of German newspaper coverage of the Olympics from 1952 to 1980, Pfister (1989) found that for female Olympic participants appearance ("beauty") was of "central importance" (Pfister, 1989 p. 11.29). Tuggle & Owen (1999) examined the amount of NBC's coverage given to female athletes at the 1996 Olympic Games and found that only women's individual events were covered extensively while the coverage of team competitions focused much more on men. Thomas and Smith (2003, p. 177) found a bigger media interest in male Paralympic athletes than females.

Female athletes with a disability are in fact subjected to multiple discrimination concerning gender, disability severity and race (cf. DePauw, 1994; DePauw & Gavron, 1995; Sherill 1993). Analyses undertaken of the 1996 Paralympics by Sherill (1997) and Schell & Duncan (1999) confirmed greater discrimination against female Paralympians than their male counterparts.

Studies on race or culture biased media coverage on disability sport are almost non-existent. According to C. A. Riley II (2005, p. xiv) "disability is the all-inclusive minority – it is completely race - and culture-blind".

Cross-cultural Differences

Researchers clearly indicate the influence of culture on the attitudes towards people with disabilities even though there was no consensus concerning the explanation of these differences (Cloerkes, 1997; Ingstad & Whyte, 1995). Indeed, Schantz & Gilbert (2001) found significant differences in coverage of the

1996 Paralympic Games in Atlanta by French and German newspapers. Overall from a cultural perspective the awareness of Paralympic sports appears to be higher in the German speaking press than in the French.

Media Coverage of the Paralympic Games

Studies relating to media coverage of the Paralympic Games are quite rare. However, Enting (1997) compared the Atlanta Paralympics coverage in a nationwide, a regional and a tabloid German newspaper (*Frankfurter Allgemeine Zeitung, Rhein-Zeitung Koblenz* and *Bildzeitung*). These newspapers offered respectively 10%, 7.5% and 0.3% of their sports pages to this event. Schell and Duncan (1999) made a content analysis of American television coverage of the Atlanta Paralympics and found that beside some empowering comments, athletes were portrayed as "victims of misfortune, as *different*, as Other" (Duncan, 1999. 27). They observed an absence of sport specific commentaries, like information about rules, comments on strategies or physical abilities. Others found that the media interest in the Paralympics is much less important than in the Olympics (Golden 2002; 2003). Contrary, to Olympic coverage, where defeats were considered as catastrophes (Duncan, 1986), the defeat of Paralympic athletes were described from patronizing perspectives (Shell & Duncan 1999).

Extraordinary performances were portrayed as heroic achievements by using the "super crip" stereotype (Shell & Duncan 1999; Goggin & Newell 2005, p. 87). According to Shapiro (1993) this "super crip" myth harms the average people with disabilities because it suggests that only heroic performances of persons with disabilities should be respected. Goggin & Newell who analyzed the 2000 Paralympics coverage in different Australian newspapers found that "there is increasing skepticism regarding received notions of disability, producing complex, contradictory media texts. However, many stories still draw on stock stereotypes of 'brave, elite athletes', 'special people', 'remarkable achievers' (Goggin & Newell, 2005, p. 86).

Schantz & Gilbert (2001) compared the print media coverage of the 1996 Atlanta Paralympics, and found that the different newspapers focused much less on sporting results than on scandals and national issues. It is interesting, when referring to the Paralympic ideals, that Schell and Duncan (1999) found, that "war and the hope for peace among people of different nationalities was a recurrent theme" and that "spectators were shown the debilitating results of war and the political barriers that may be dissolved through friendly sport competition" (p.43).

Zeros or Heroes, or Is There an in-between?

As the review of the research literature shows, there are still two dominating attitudes in the media towards Paralympic sports: either to ignore more or less these sport events or to construe the myth of the supercrip, the freaky cyborg or the hero who overcame his terrible fate.

Despite the claim of the official representatives from the International Paralympic Committee and the International Committee, that the Paralympic Games and the Olympic Games are parallel Games, there is a huge gap in between these events. The symbolic and financial capital of the Olympic Games is enormous and cannot be compared with the Paralympic Games. The Olympics are selling a dream which corresponds to the ideals of today's mass culture: to be fit, fine-looking, and famous.

Both movements however, create heroes - the Olympic hero is mostly a dramatic creation of the sporting contest, the Paralympic hero is a product of the real life drama. The first-one generates envy or offers an identification model, the second-one calls for admiration or engenders pity. The role model potential of the disabled hero has to be considered with care. The common sense argument, that Paralympic athletes serve the empowerment of the community of people with disabilities is an ambiguous one. Indeed, the Paralympics show the prowess these people are able to achieve, but at the same time they make believe, that every person with disabilities can achieve success provided he or she is dedicated and hardworking enough. Many people with disabilities, however, have to struggle enormously in order to achieve daily routines like dressing, shopping, or travelling. The percentage of those able and willing to practice any sport is rather marginal. The success of a few disadvantaged athletes hides the failure of the great majorities who try but fail (Sage, 1990; Eitzen, 2009).

What sportswomen and men with disabilities probably need is media coverage in between the zero and the hero, a coverage which respects them as full and equal members of the sporting community. They do not need pity, neither heroic stories based on their disabilities; they need the right to play sports, an accessible sport world, and respect for their sporting performances. By describing and showing a realistic and respectful picture of the sport activities of people with disabilities, the media could help to challenge obsolete cultural norms and to prepare an inclusive sporting world, respecting the broad diversity of the physiques and abilities of humans. The chapterin this important book on marginalization and disability will hopefully add to the literature in this area and engender further research and understanding of the media – Paralympic – disability conundrum.

References

Albright, A. C. (1997). *Choreographing difference. The body and identity in contemporary dance. H*anover, NH: Wesleyan University Press.

Baudrillard, J. (1991, March 29). La guerre du Golfe n'a pas eu lieu. *Libération.*

Becker, p. (1983). Sport in den Massenmedien. *Sportwissenschaft 13* (1), 24-45.

Bell, A. (1991). *The language of news media.* Oxford, UK, Cambridge MA: Blackwell.

Berelson, B. (1960). Communication and public opinion. In W. Schramm (Ed.), *Mass communications* (pp. 527-543). Urbana: University of Illinois Press.

Berghaus, M. (1999). Wie Massenmedien wirken. *Rundfunk und Fernsehen 47* (2), 181-199.

Bette, K. H. (1999). *Systemtheorie und Sport.* Frankfurt a. M.: Suhrkamp.

Blinde, E. M., & McCallister, S. G. (1999). Women, disability, and sport and physical activity: The intersection of gender and disability dynamics. *Research Quarterly for Exercise and Sport, 70,* 303-312.

Borcila, A. (2000). Nationalizing the Olympics around and away from "vulnerable" bodies of women: The NBC coverage of the 1996 Olympics and some moments after. *Journal ofSport and Social Issues, 24* (2), 118-147.

Bourdieu, P. (1994). Les Jeux Olympiques. Programme pour une analyse. *Actes de la Recherche en Sciences Sociales, 103,* 102-103.

Bourdieu, P. (1996). *Sur la télévision.* Paris: Liber.

Chambre des Communes (1988). *Pas de nouvelles, mauvaises nouvelles.* Premier rapport du Comité permanent de la condition des personnes handicapées. Ottawa: Chambre des Communes.

Cloerkes, G. (1997). *Soziologie der Behinderten.* Heidelberg: Schindle.

Clogston, J. S. (1994). Disability coverage in American newspapers. In J. A. Nelson (Ed.), *The disabled, the media, and the information age* (pp. 45-53). Westport, CN: Greenwood Press.

Coakley, Jay J. (1994) *Sport in society. Issues and controversies.* St. Louis: Mosby

Cole, C. (1999 August, 27). Faster, higher, poorer. N*ational Post*, Canada.

Dearing, J. W., Rogers, E. M. (1996). *Agenda setting.* London: Sage.

DePauw, K. (1997). The (in)visibility of disability: Cultural contexts and sporting bodies. *Quest, 49,* 416-430.

DePauw, K. (2000). Social‑Cultural Context of Disability: Implications for Scientific Inquiry and Professional Preparation. *Quest 52,* 358-368.

DePauw, K. P. (1997). The (In)Visibility of DisAbility: Cultural contexts and "sporting bodies". *Quest, 49,* 416-430.

DePauw, K., & Gavron, S. (1995). *Disability and sport.* Champaign: Human Kinetics.

Donsbach, W. (1991). *Medienwirkung trotz Selektion. Einflußfaktoren auf die Zuwendung zu Zeitungsinhalten.* Köln: Böhlauer.

Donsbach, W. (1992). Die Selektivität der Rezipienten. Faktoren, die die Zuwendung zu Zeitungsinhalten beeinflussen. In W. Schulz (Ed.), *Medienwirkungen. Einflüsse von Presse Radio und Fernsehen auf Individuen und Gesellschaft* (pp. 25-71). Weinheim: VCH.

Duhamel, A. (1985). *Le complexe d'Astérix.* Paris: Gallimard.

Dummer, G. M. (1998). Media coverage of disability sport.*Palaestra, 14* (4), 56.

Duncan, M. C. (1986). A hermeneutic of spectator sport: The 1976 and 1984 Olympic Games. *Quest, 38,* 50-77.

Duncan, M. C. (1990). Sports photographs and sexual difference. The images of women and men in the 1984 and 1988 Olympic Games. S*ociology of Sport Journal, 7,* 22-43.

Duncan, M. C.; Messner, M., & Williams, L. (1991). *Coverage of women's sports in four daily newspapers.* Edited by W. Wayne. Los Angeles: AAF publications. Retrieved January 27, 2000 from the World Wide Web: http://www.   AAFLA.org/Publications/-ResearchReports/ResearchReport1_.htm.

Eastman, S. T. & Billings, A. (2000). Sportcasting and sports reporting. The power of the gender bias. J*ournal of Sport& Social Issues, 24* (2), 192-213.

Eco, U. (1997). *Cinque scritti morali.* Milano: Bompiani.

Eilders, C. (1997). *Nachrichtenfaktoren und Rezeption. Eine empirische Analyse zur Auswahl und Verarbeitung politischer Information.* Opladen: Westdeutscher Verlag.

Eitzen, S. D. (2009). *Fair and Foul. Beyond Myths and Paradoxes of Sport.* Lanham: Rowman & Littlefield.

Elias, N. & Dunning E. (1970). The quest of excitement in unexciting societies. In G. Lüschen (ed.). *The cross-cultural analysis of sport and games* (pp. 31-51). Champaign, IL: Stipes.

Enting, B. (1997). Die Berichterstattung über die Paralympics 1996 in Atlanta - dargestellt in ausgewählten Printmedien. Unpublished master's thesis, Sport University Cologne, Köln, Germany.

Erbring, L., Goldenberg, E., & Miller, A. (1980). Front pages news and real world cues: A New Look at Agenda-Setting by the Media. *American Journal of Political Science, 24* (1), pp- 19-49.

Farnall, O. & K. A. Smith (1999). Reactions to people with disabilities: Personal contact versus viewing of specific media portrayals. *Journalism and Mass Communication Quarterly, 76* (4), 659-672.

Fiske, J. (1993). *Power plays, power works.* London: Verso.

Foucault, M. (1961). *Histoire de la folie à l'âge classique.* Paris: Gallimard.

Früh, W. (1994). *Realitätsvermittlung durch Massenmedien. Die permanente Transformation der Wirklichkeit.* Opladen: Westdeutscher Verlag.

Galtung, J., & Ruge, H. (1965). The structure of foreign news. Journal of Peace Research, 2, 64-91.

Gebauer, G. (1994). Le nouveau nationalisme sportif. *Actes de la Recherche en Sciences Sociales, 103,* 104-107.

Génolini, J.P. (1995). L'expression euphémique du handicap mental dans les messages de presse sur le sport. *Revue Européenne du Handicap Mental, 2* (8), 54-63.

Gill, C. J. (1994). Questioning continuum. In B. Shaw (Ed.), *The ragged edge: The disability experience from the pages of the first fifteen years of The Disability Rag* (pp. 42-49). Louisville, KY: Avocado Press.

Goggin, G. & Newell, C. (2005). *Disability in Australia: Exposing a Social Apartheid.* Sydney: UNSW Press.

Golden, A. (2003). An Analysis of the Dissimilar Coverage of the 2002 Olympics and Paralympics: Frenzied Pack Journalism versus the Empty Press Room. *Disability Studies Quarterly 23,* (3/4) (www.dsq-sds.org).

Golden, A. (2002). An Analysis of the Dissimilar Coverage of the 2002 Olympics and Paralympics: Frenzied Pack Journalism Versus the Empty Press Room. Media& Disability Interest Group, Association for Education in Journalism and Mass Communication Annual Meeting, Miami, Fl.

Greenberg, B. S. & J. S. Brand (1994). Minorities and the mass media: 1970 to 1990. In J. Bryant & D. Zillmann (Eds.), *Media Effects: Advances in Theory and Research* (pp. 273-314). Hillsdale NJ: L. Erlbaum.

Guttmann, A. (1996). *The erotics in sport.* New York: Columbia University Press.

Guttmann, L. (1949). The second national Stoke Mandeville Games of the paralysed. *The Cord,* 3, 24.

Guttmann, L. (1979). *Sport für Körperbehinderte* [Textbook of Sport for the Disabled]. München: Urban& Schwarzenberg.

Hackforth, J. (1988). Publizistische Wirkungsforschung: Ansätze, Analysen und Analogien. In J. Hackforth (Ed.), *Sportmedien und Mediensport* (pp. 15-33). Berlin: Vistas.

Hackforth, J. (1994). Behindertensport in den Medien. In: Behinderten-Sportverband Nordrhein-Westfalen (Hrsg.). *Behindertensport : Sein Stellenwert in der Arbeitswelt und Gesellschaft.* Duisburg: BSVNW, pp. 46-48.

Hall, S. (1997). The spectacle of the 'other'. In S. Hall (Ed.). *Representation. Cultural representations and signifying practices* (pp. 223- 290). London: Sage

Haller, B. (2000). If they limp, they lead? News representations and the hierarchy of disability images. In D. Braithwaite & T. Thompson, (Eds.), *Handbook of Communication and People with Disabilities* (pp. 273-288). Mahwah, NJ: Lawrence Erlbaum Associates.

Hardin, M. (2003). Marketing the acceptably athletic image: Wheelchair athletes, sport-related advertising and capitalist hegemony. *Disability Studies Quarterly, 23*(1), 108-125.

Hardin, M. M. & Hardin, B. (2004). The 'Supercrip' in sport media: Wheelchair athletes discuss hegemony's disabled hero. *sosol 7*. Retrieved January 10, 2005 from: http://physed.otago.ac.nz/sosol/v7i1/ v7i1_1.html.

Hiestand, M. (July 25, 2000). Paralympics online to test live market. U*S Today,* C.9.

Holicki, S. (1993). *Pressefoto und Pressetext im Wirkungsvergleich. Eine experimentelle Untersuchung am Beispiel von Politikerdarstellungen.* München: Fischer.

Horkheimer, M., & Adorno, Th. W. (1989 [1947]). *Dialektik der Aufklärung. Philosophische Fragmente.* Leipzig: Reclam.

Howe, D. (2008). From Inside the Newsroom: Paralympic Media and the "Production" of Elite Disability. *International Review for the Sociology of Sport, 43* (2), 135150.

Ingstad, B. & Whyte, S. R. (1995). *Disability and culture.* Berkley: University of California Press.

International Olympic Committee (1996). O*lympic charter.* Lausanne: I. O. C.

International Paralympic Committee (2000). *IPC constitution.* Retrieved February 1st, 2000 from the World Wide Web: http://www.paralympic.org

Internenettes (Eds.) (2000). *Représentations des femmes dans la vie politique française.* Retrieved April 2nd, 2000 from the World Wide Web: http://www.internenettes.fr/femmes/politique.html

Jamieson, K. H., Campbell, K. K. (1997). *The interplay of influence. News, advertising, politics, and the mass media. Belmont,* 4th edition. CA: Wadsworth.

Jones, R., Murell, A. J. & Jackson J. (1999). Pretty versus powerful in the sports pages. *Journal of Sport& Social Issues, 23* (2), 183-192.

Kauer, O., & Bös, K. (1998). *Behindertensport in den Medien. A*achen: Meyer & Meyer:

Keller, C. E., Hallahan, D. P., McShane, E. A., Crowley, E. P., & Blandford, B. J. (1990). The coverage of persons with disabilities in American newspapers. The Journal of Special Education, 24 (3), 271-282.

Kellner, D. (1995). Media culture- Cultural studies, identity and politics between the modern and the postmodern. London: Routledge.

Kepplinger, M. H. (1986). Begriffe und Modelle langfristiger Medienwirkung. In W. A. Mahle (Ed.), Langfristige Medienwirkung (pp. 27-38). Berlin: Wissenschaftsverlag Volker Spiess.

Klapper, J. T. (1960). The effects of mass Communication. Glencoe, Ill.: Free Press.

Krüger, A. (1993). Cui bono? Die Rolle des Sports in den Massenmedien. In A. Krüger, & A., Scharenberg (Eds.), Wie die Medien den Sport aufbereiten - Ausgewählte Aspekte der Sportpublizistik (pp. 24-63). Berlin: Tischler.

Kuhn, R. (1995). The media in France. London: Routledge.

Lachal, R.-C. (1990a). La presse française et les personnes handicapées de 1977 à 1988. In Institut de l'Enfance et de la Famille (Ed.), Handicap, famille et société (pp. 39-44). Paris: IDEF.

Lachal, R.-C. (1990b). Les personnes handicapées vues par la presse régionale française. Constantes et évolutions de 1977 à 1988. Handicaps et Inadaptations - Les Cahiers du CTNERHI, 51/52, 1-29.

Lazarsfeld, P. F., & Merton, R. K. (1948). Mass communication, popular taste and organized social action. In L. Bryson (Ed.), Communication of ideas (pp. 95-118). New York: Harper & Bros.

Lazarsfeld, P. F., Berelseon, B., & Gaudet, H. (1968). The people's choice (3rd ed.). New York: Columbia University Press.

Levine, S. (2000). Narrowing the perception gap. The Quill, 88 (3), 35.

Longmore, P. K. (1985). Screening stereotypes: Images of disabled people. Social Policy, 16 (1), 31-37.

Luebke, B. (1989). Out of focus. Images of women and men in the newspaper photographs. Sex Roles, 20 (3-4), 121-133.

Luhmann, N. (1996). Die Realität der Massenmedien (2nd ed.). Opladen: Westdeutscher Verlag.

Lyotard, J.-F. (1983). Le différend. Paris: Editions de Minuit.

Maguire, J. (1993). Globalization, sport development and the media/sport production complex. Sport Science Review, 2 (1), 29-47.

McCombs, M. (1994). News influence on our pictures of the world. In J. Bryant, & D. Zillmann (Eds.), Media effects. Advances in theory and research (pp. 1- 16). Hillsdale, NJ: Lawrence Erlbaum.

McQuail, D. (1993). Mass Communication Theory. London, Thousand Oaks, New Dehli.

Merten, K. (1995). Inhaltsanalyse. Opladen: Westdeutscher Verlag.

Münch, R. (1993). Die Kultur der Moderne. Band2: Ihre Entwicklung in Frankreich und Deutschland. Frankfurt a. M.: Suhrkamp.

Nelson, J. A. (1994). Broken Images: Portrayals of those with disabilities in American media. In J. A. Nelson (Ed.), The disabled, the media, and the information age (pp. 1-17). Westport, CN: Greenwood Press.

Noelle-Neumann, E. (1994). Wirkung der Massenmedien auf die Meinungsbildung. In E. Noelle-Neumann, W. Schulz, & J. Wilke (Eds.),

Publizistik, Massenkommunikation (pp. 518-571). Frankfurt a. M.: Fischer.

Oakes, P. J., Haslam, A., & J. C. Turner (1994). S*tereotyping and social reality.* Cambridge, MA: Blackwell.

Oehmichen, E. (1991). Sport im Alltag - Sport im Fernsehen. *Media Perspektiven, 11,* 744-758.

Pappous, A., Marcellini, A., & Léséleuc, E. de (2011). Contested issues in research on the media coverage of feamle Paralympic athletes. *Sport in Society,* 14(9), 1182-1191.

Peltu, M. (1985). The role of communication media. In H. Ottway, & M. Peltu (Eds.), *Regulating industrial risks: Science, hazards and public protection* (pp. 128-148). London.

Pfister, G. (1987). Women in the Olympics (1952-1980): An analysis of German newspapers (beauty vs. gold medals). In *The Olympic movement and the mass media* (pp. 11.27–11.37). Calgary: Hurford.

Riggs, K. E., Eastman, S. T., & Golobic, T. S. (1993). Manufactured conflict in the 1992 Olympics: the discourse of television and politics. *Critical Studies in Mass Communication, 10* (3), 253-272.

Riley II, C. A. (2005). *Disability and the Media.Prescriptions for Change.* Hanover, London: University Press of New England.

Robertson, R. (1992). *Globalization: social theory and global culture.* London: Sage.

Rowe, D. (1999). *Sport, culture and the media. The untruly trinity.* Buckingham, PH: Open University Press.

Sage, G. H. (1990).*Power and Ideology in American Sport: A Critical Perspective. Champaign*, Ill.: Human Kinetics.

Sandfort, L. (1982). Medien-Manifest. Forderung behinderter an die Medien. In: H. J. Kagelmann & R. Zimmermann (Eds.). *Massenmedien und Behinderte. Im besten Falle Mitleid?* Weinheim, Basel: Beltz Verlag,.

Schantz, O. (1999). La mise en scène du corps extraordinaire - Freak show ou implication éthique de l'esthétique. In Centre de Recherche en Education Corporelle (Ed.). *La danse, une culture en mouvement* (pp. 67-74). Strasbourg : UMB.

Schantz, O., & Alberto, C. (1999). Coping strategies of Paralympic athletes."In *12° Congreso Mundial de Actividad Fisica Adaptada - COMAFA '99, 4-8 de Mayo de 1999 Barcelona - Lleida.* Resumenes. Barcelona: Institut Nacional d'educació Física de Catalunya, pp. 95-96.

Schantz, O. J. & Gilbert, K. (2001). An ideal misconstrued: Newspaper coverage of the Atlanta Paralympic Games in France and Germany. *Sociology of Sport Journal 18*, 69-94.

Schantz, O. J. & Gilbert, K. (2008). French and German Newspaper Coverage oft he 1996 Atlanta Paralympic Games. In K. Gilbert & O. J. Schantz (Eds.). The Paralympic Games. Empowerment or Side Show? (pp. 34-56). Maidenhead: Meyer& Meyer.

Schantz, O., & Marty, C. (1995). The French press and sport for people with handicapping conditions. In I. Morisbak, P. E. Jørgensen (Eds.) *Quality of live through adapted physical activity* (pp. 72-79). Oslo: Hamtrykk.

Schell, L. A. & Duncan, M. (1999). A Content Analysis of CBS's Coverage of the 1996 Paralympic Games. *Adapted Physical Activity Quarterly, 16,* 2747.

Schell, L. A., & Duncan, M. C. (1999). A content analysis of CBS's coverage of the 1996 Paralympic Games. *Adapted Physical Activity Quarterly, 16* (1), pp. 27-47.

Schimanski, M. (1994). Behindertensport in der deutschen und amerikanischen Tagespresse 1984-1992. Unter besonderer Berücksichtigung der Paralympics. Eine Analyse anhand ausgewählter Printmedien. Unpublished master's thesis, Sport University Cologne, Köln, Germany.

Scholz, M. (2010). *Presse und Behinderung.* Wiesbaden: Verlag für Sozialwissenschaften.

Schönbach, K. (1992). Transaktionale Modelle der Medienwirkung: Stand der Forschung. In W. Schulz (Ed.), *Medienwirkungen. Einflüsse von Presse Radio und Fernsehen auf Individuen und Gesellschaft* (pp. 109-120). Weinheim: VCH.

Segrave, J. O. (1988). Toward a definition of Olympism. In J. O. Segrave & D. Chu (Eds.). *The Olympic Games in transition* (pp. 149-161). Champaign, IL: Human Kinetics.

Shapiro, J. P. (1993). *No pity: People with disabilities forging a new civil rights movement.* New York: Times Books.

Sherill, C. (1993). Women with disabilities. In G. Cohen (Ed.), *Women in sport: Issues and controversies* (pp. 238-248). Newbury Park, CA: Sage.

Sherill, C. (1997). Paralympic Games 1996: Feminist and other concerns: What's your excuse? *Palestra, 13,* 32-38.

Silva, C. F. & Howe, D. P. (2012). The (In)validity of Supercrip Representation of Paralympian Athletes, *Journal of Sport& Social Issues* (online first January 26), 2012, 1-21.

Smith, A. & Thomas, N. (2005). The "inclusion" of elite athletes with disabilities in the 2002 Manchester Commonwealth Games: an exploratory analysis of British newspaper coverage. *Sport, Education and Society, 10* (1), 49-67.

Stautner, B. K. (1989). *Abweichung - Behinderung - Sport in der modernen Gesellschaft. Eine Bestandsaufnahme und systemtheoretische Neuformulierung.* Unpublished doctoral dissertation. Julius-Maximilians University, Würzburg.

Sutton, J. (Jan 5, 1998). Sponsors shy away from Paralympic Games. Marketing News, 32 (1), 21-22.

Thomas, N. & Smith, A. (2003). Preoccupied with Able - Bodiedness? An Analysis of the British Media Coverage of the 2000 Paralympics Games. *Adapted Physical Activity Quarterly, 20,* 166-181.

Tuggle, C. A. & Owen, A. (1999). A descriptive analysis of the centennial Olympics: the 'Games of the Women'? *Journal of Sport and Social Issues, 23* (2), 171-182.

Turner, B. S. (1998). Foreword.. In W. Seymour, *Remaking the Body. Rehabilitation and Change* (v-viii). St Leonards: Allen & Unwin.

Urquhart, J. & Crossman, J. (1999). The Globe and Mail coverage of the winter Olympic Games. J*ournal of Sport& Social Issues, 23* (2), 193-202.

Wann, D. L., Schrader, M. P., Allison, J. A. & McGeorge K. K. (1998). The inequitable newspaper coverage of men's and women's athletics at small, medium, and large universities. *Journal of Sport& Social Issues, 22* (1), 79-87.

Waxman, B. F. (1994). It's time to politicize our sexual oppression. In B. Shaw (Ed.), *The ragged edge: The disability experience from the pages of the first fifteen years of The Disability Rag* (pp. 82-87). Louisville, KY: Avocado Press.

White, D., M. (1950). The »Gatekeeper«: A case study in the selection of news. *Journalism Quarterly, 27,* 383-390.

Wilke, J. (1994). Presse. In E. Noelle-Neumann, W. Schulz, & J. Wilke (Eds.), *Publizistik, Massenkommunikation* (pp. 382-417). Frankfurt a. M.: Fischer.

Woodill, G. (1994). The social semiotics of disability. In M. H. Rioux & M. Bach (Eds.). D*isability is not measles. New research paradigms in disability* (pp. 201-226). North York, Ontario: Roeher.

Yoshida, R. K., Wasilewski, L., & Friedman, D. L. (1990). Recent newspaper coverage about persons with disabilities. *Exceptional children, 56,* 418-423.

Zola, I. K. (1985). Depictions of disability – Metaphor, message, and medium in the media: A research and political agenda. *The Social Science Journal, 22* (4), 5-17.

Chapter 4: Cultural Perspectives on Mental Health and Community Based Rehabilitation in Sri Lanka

Rachel Tribe

Introduction

Models of disability have on occasions been based rather heavily on pre conceived notions of physical or mental ability which could be viewed as both narrow and reductionist and which appear to assume that there are universal 'norms' which can be measured regardless of context or individualism. These notions contained assumptions including that of a medical model of disability being the predominant and only model. These early models often failed to account for a wide range of factors which will effect the way individuals, cultures and societies construct the notion of disability. As more sophisticated and complex models have developed including the social and empowerment models which have taken into account important variables and mediating factors which include but are not limited to individual, societal and cultural meanings, context, identity and socio-cultural or political perspectives, as well as a temporalperspective. These have all allowed a richer fuller model of disability to emerge which more accurately reflects the lived experiences of people with a range of disabilities.(For a full discussion of these issues see chapter 2 of this volume). This discussion will not be reiterated further here. Although it is perhaps important to note that learning disability, a label which in itself is contested by a number of service users and service user groups, but is widely used by statutory services (Goodley, 2001) illustrates the role of socio-cultural political and cultural constructions in definitions within one specific cultural context, that of Britain. Whilst coverage by the British media TV Channel 4 in 2012 on the Para-Olympics where they have consistently used the term super-humans to describe the Para - Olympians perhaps also illustrates the way language and culture can play a part in definingand constructingnotions of disability.

Whilst mental health and psychological well–being has sometimes been excluded from formulations relating to definitions of disability, it is claimed that twenty five per cent of the population will suffer from mental health issues during a one year period (Mental Health Foundation, 2012)with 1:6 people experiencing mental health issues at any given time (Office for National Statistic Psychiatric Morbidity report, 2001). The disabling effects of this can be numerous and may include social deprivation, the inability to maintain relationships, substance misuse, self harm and homelessness. The National Institute for Mental Health in the USA have constructed a measure of disability adjusted life years (DALYS) for those suffering from severe mental illness, which includes years lost to illness, disability or premature death, these figures are a grave cause for concern. Therefore the effects can be disabling both for the individual, their families, work place and the multiple communities of which we are all a part. Mental health issues are still assigned a stigma by some people which can lead to marginalisation and discrimination (Mind, 2011; Royal College of Psychiatrists, 2003; Dept of Health Information Centre, 2011).

As mentioned earlier, constructions of what constitutes disabilities and mental health across cultures may differ and may well reflect the values held within that culture or sub culture about mental health or disability. For example western notions of good mental health carry positivist notions of what comprises good mental health and may not be generalizable outside western countries as is often unquestioningly assumed by those located in the west (Patel, 2004)."Summerfield (2002: 248) writing about the manuals used to diagnose mental illness developed in the USA and Europe claims that the:"Diagnostic Statistical Manual (DSM) and International Classifications of Diseases (ICD) are not, as some imagine, atheoretical and purely descriptive nosologies with universal validity. They are western cultural documents, carrying ontological notions of what constitutes a real disorder, epistemological ideas about what counts as scientific evidence, and methodological ideas as to how research should be conducted."If a patient in the USA presents with a set of symptoms which do not match a diagnosis in the DSM, they can not get treatment under their health insurance and a psychiatrist or psychologist may not be allowed to treat them. Therefore the DSM is a highly political document with lobbyists advocating on a number of fronts for a particular diagnosis to be included. It is updated every few years with some new categorisations added and some left out. It also reflects socio-cultural mores, for example homosexuality was contained and viewed as an illness in earlier versions.

How we define poor mental health and well-being will always be culturally located and western notions may not adequately account for cultural differences in relation to the positioning and presentation of emotional distress (Fernando, 2011). This chapter will look at a range of community based well-being or mental health rehabilitation projects located in Sri Lanka. We have taken a position that mental health is located within a matrix of factors and is not a unitary entity. In Sri Lanka, as in most of the world, mental illness is frequently viewed as stigmatising (Samarasekera et al, 2012) negatively and may be viewed as a form of disability. This chapter will look at a number of community based rehabilitation projects which we ran in Sri Lanka.

The author was working with a team of people of Sri Lankan heritage, weconsidered and valued the rich sources of support and meaningin relation to well being and health found in most cultures and in this context within Sri Lanka.

We reflected upon how these can be undermined by an insistence onapplying western ideas uncritically which can inadvertently undermine conventional cultural wisdom andsystems. With approximately 30 psychiatrists and a handful of psychologists working in Sri Lanka working in a traditional western individually based 'treatment' model was never going to be feasible even if this was the model of choice. Some Sri Lankan peoplemayview having mental health concerns as very frightening. As the following quote in relation to someone from Sri Lanka who had recently moved to the UK illustrates, notions of good mental health are likely to be partly culturally defined."One of the clients [...] had made an [...] counselling appointment in the UK, but in Sri Lanka actually mental means you are really mad. So when her brother saw that appointment obviously he thought she's mental. [And] she was just scared about the appointment, she started to cry, she asked us: am I mental? You know seeing me, and I said like: no, mental health [...] covers many different meanings so I had to explain like it doesn't mean like you're mental actually, don't worry."

Sri Lanka

A map showing the location of Sri Lanka is shown in Fig 1. There was a civil war of 26 years duration in Sri Lanka, which was won militarily by the Sri Lanka army in May 2009. The civil war was between the Tamil militants, known as the Liberation Tigers of Tamil Eelam (LTTE), or more colloquially the Tamil Tigers, were fighting against the Sri Lankan army for control of the north-east with the aim of creating an autonomous Tamil state there. Human rights violations were recorded by both sides in the civil war (Human Rights Watch, 2009). As a result of military action and violence on both sides, approximately 70,000 men, women and children from all the ethnic groups lost their lives during the war (Reuters 2009In addition concerns about trust and secrecy may become functional strategies in a civil war situation (Tribe, 2007). Some people may be fearful of trusting anyone, and normal social bonds and community life may have been challengedand fragmentedfor some people (Somasandaram, 2007).

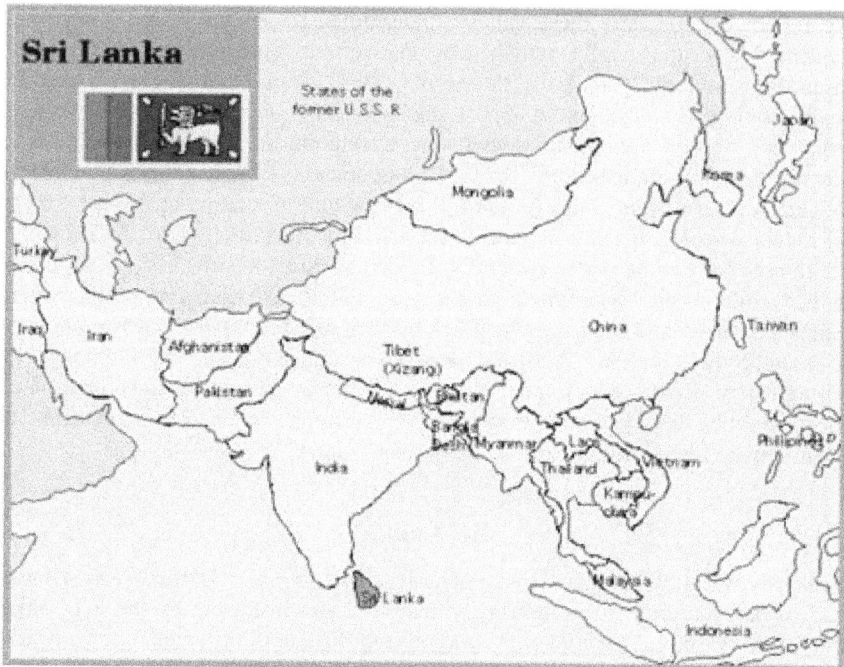

Fig 1. Showing location of Sri Lanka.

Approximately 1.8 million people were uprooted by the civil war (UNHCR, 2009) and many people fled overseas. Weerackody & Fernando (2009) reported that many of those who were internally displaced had been subjected to repeated trauma, loss and bereavement over many years. The south Asian tsunami of December 2004also caused considerable damage to three quarters of the country's coastline and 230,000 people lost family members, homes, property and their livelihoods (Save the Children Fund, 2006). In addition in January 2011, the east of Sri Lanka suffered from serious flooding, with 127,000 people displaced from their homes (UN, 2011) as shown in fig 2. Therefore many Sri Lankans have therefore lived through extremely stressful times.

Traumatic events, civil war and forced displacement, can affect people and the communities they are part of, in any number of ways. They may face a whole series of challenges, which may include practical and psychological losses and subsequent well-being may be affected. Our perspective is that well being as being embedded in a matrix of contextual factors, which may include familial, community, spiritual, cultural, and socio-political issues, as well as individual, familial and cultural support and meaning-making systems (Tribe, 2004). Therefore working exclusively with 'traumatised' individuals may not be the best way forward in helping a community rebuild itself, its sense of identity and to develop resilience and a shared future.

Issues of justice, fairness and socio-political considerations may also play a role in how an individual and the wider community in Sri Lanka construes and processes the effects of civil war, the tsunami (December 2004) and the flooding in early 2011. Weerackody & Fernando (2011) have published details of the research on mental health and well-being they conducted in four disparate locations in Sri Lanka and have stressed the need to consider the entire community and the importance of supporting the natural resilience found within them. This is in line with the Inter-Agency Standing Committee (IASC, 2007) guidelines on Mental Health and Psychosocial Support in Emergency Settings.

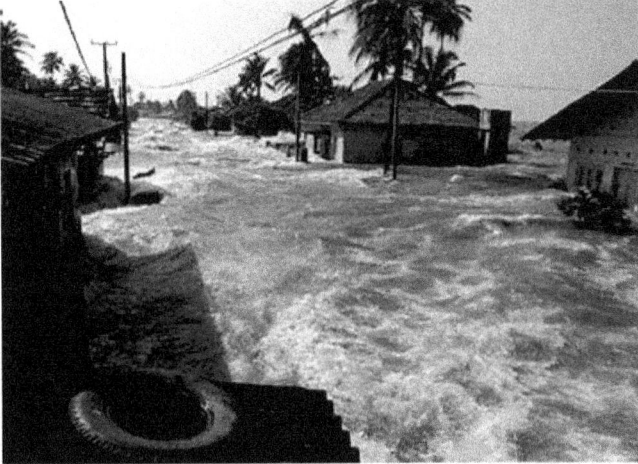

Fig 2. Flooding In East Sri Lanka, causing severe displacement of people from their homes (UN,2011).

This chapter will next consider the possible effects on psychological wellbeing and what may be the most appropriate paradigms and descriptors to consider and use when describing these effects. These need to be culturally respectful, as well as meaningful and useful to survivors of traumatic events, war, conflict and forced migration, where ever they may be living. As Fernando (2010) working in Sri Lanka has noted individualised therapy may not be the most helpful way forward, as it can be viewed as stigmatising and can inadvertently undermine cultural sources of healing and resources which have always been used to deal with distress. Community interventions and group or family based collaborations may be more appropriate, examples of these interventions in Sri Lanka can be located in Somasundaram & Sivayokan (2000), Tribe &De Silva (1999); Tribe (2004); Weerackody & Fernando (2011). The literature on trauma and Post Traumatic Stress Disorder (PTSD) and the major arguments on this contested topic will be briefly summarised, as well as that on resilience.

Effects of War, Civil Conflict and Displacement

Definitions and Descriptors Used

There is no doubt that war, civil conflict, displacement and becoming an internal refugee or internally displaced person and living through traumatic events are not conducive to good psychological health at the individual, family and community level as outlined in diagram 1 (WHO, 2000). Whether or not this is best described in terms of basic human and community reactions to abnormal and adverse events and as distress rather than as an individualised diagnosable mental illness particularly in relation to Post Traumatic Stress Disorder (PTSD) using a western diagnostic system is contested. A complete review of this debate is unfortunately outside the scope of this chapter and the interested reader is referred to Summerfield, (2001); Bracken & Petty (1999); Rousseau & Measham, (2007); de Silva, (1999).

Weerackody & Fernando (2011) working in Sri Lanka have recommended the following policies in areas affected by conflict and disaster; the strengthening of human and social capital, restoring incomes and livelihoods, reducing feelings of insecurity, protecting vulnerable people, enabling displaced people to return to what they consider their 'homes' as soon as possible, reducing alcohol and drug use, improving social cohesion and mutual support. There have frequently been assumptions made that people who have lived through traumatic events must be psychologically damaged by them and the term PTSD has often been over-used and used uncritically (Summerfield, 2001). Although more recent research has started to question this assumption and has noted the considerable resilience shown by individuals and communities at such times (Bonanno, 2004; Rousseau, & Measham, 2007) who may not present with psychological distress or PTSD in the longer term. Apart from issues about the appropriateness of applying western bio medical categories to cultures uncritically (Bracken & Petty, 1999). In a world which appears to be increasingly reliant on labelling, positivist measurement and reductionism this may be understandable particularly when being given a diagnosis of PTSD can lead the individual bearer to obtain accessto support or services. Also a mental health professional is often distressed by the experience of the individual and community and being able to offer something i.e. a diagnosis which may appear to help the individual who has survived such traumatic eventsin some way, may feel important to them. On the other hand obtaining a diagnosis can be stigmatising for the individual and their family (Byrne, 2000). Internal displacement or refugee status and forced migration were the result of the conflict and tsunami for many people in Sri Lanka.

Some individuals and communities may suffer from trauma related issues and some may develop PTSD as many have been through very difficulttimes and may require psychological and practical support, at some point in the process or afterwards. How adaptive dilemmas or difficulties are labelled and the paradigms used to offer help are important as they may define what and how resources are allocated and who subsequently receives help. In addition Individuals and communities may be more concerned about lack of housing, security, schooling and employment and their future lives rather than their current mental state (Summerfield, 2001; Somasundaram, & Sivayokan, 2000). Weerackody& Fernando (2011) have stressed the need for community based mental health services in rural communitiesin Sri Lanka. A label of PTSD, a condition diagnosed by a psychiatrist and a mental health issue can be interpreted by survivors in many different ways, some of which will be culturally defined. All cultures contain a range of views about mental health relating to causes, treatment, sources of help and subsequent labelling. For example, a diagnosis may be seen as something very serious which means that an individual person is viewed as damaged in some way or it may be used as a functional strategy for the individual to access resources. It was to minimise any potential labelling or stigma for any individual who was traumatised or suffering from psychological difficulties that we decided that community based rehabilitation was the most helpful way forward. Community based rehabilitation can provide a normalising function and can also ensure that this is based on what a community requires at that particular time. Mental health services operate in a political socio-cultural context and this may also define to some degree how they are structured and used (Fernando, 2003; Weerackody & Fernando, 2011; Tribe, 2007). Those who uncritically expect to find a population who are traumatised may find just that, and those who do not expect to find that, may similarly find what they are looking for, for example Summerfield (1999) as McNamee & Gergen (1992) write;

> "We not only bear languages that furnish the rationale for our looking, but also vocabularies of description and explanation for what is observed. Thus, we confront life situations with codes in hand, fore-structures of understanding which themselves suggest how we are to sortthe problematic from the precious". (McNamee & Gergen, 1992, p.1)

Equally it would be unethical to deny individual help to traumatised individuals who require it. There are likely to be some individuals who suffer from a range of traumatic reactions which will include PTSD, but this will be a percentage of the population, not the entire population. Therefore the issue is what are the sources of healing, cultural traditions, religious or spiritual practices which people use intimes of difficulty, as well as how far are the concepts and methods of western psychiatry, diagnosis and labelling using individualised biomedical notions of ill or mental health are appropriate to radically different cultures and contexts. It appears that both traditional and cultural practices which may combine with elements of western psychological theory in an equal but constructive partnership may be considered one way forward. In reality this may need careful and considered discussion as resource and power differentials can be present. There may well be people who would also benefit from individual assistance and it has been suggested that health pluralism which accepts a range of models may be a helpful way forward (Tribe, 2007). In addition complex ecological emergencies or traumatic events which an entire country experiences such as a civil war may affect communities at the family, community and societal level and it may be more helpful to take a systemic perspective. Somasundaram (2010) has written about the notion of collective trauma where a society or communities of people become traumatised and fail to function as successfully as they had done previously. All parts of a community can be affected, with family relationships, social structures, peer groups and social structures becoming fragmented and distorted as depicted in Diagram 1

Adverse Effects of Political Violence and Displacement on Individuals, Families and Communities (Tribe, 2009 adapted from Miller & Rasco, 2004)

Political Conflict

Loss of social networks, leading to social isolation

Community Well-being

Loss of trust, dissolution of communal ties and institutions, loss of community through displacement

D IS P L A C E M E N T

Loss of social roles and role related activities

Unemployment, poverty-related stressors

Loss of environmental mastery,

Discrimination

Separation from loved ones, concern for their welfare

Intergenerational differences in rates of acculturation

The Psychological Effects of Political Conflict and displacement on individuals, Families, and communities

Family Well-being

Increased family tension and conflict, grief and disorganisation resulting from death or disappearance of family members, strain on families of individual family members' own distress

Individual Well-being

Conflict-related trauma, traumatic grief, depression, anxiety due to displacement-related stressors, indigenous expressions of distress, resilience

Post-displacement Stressors not directly Related to Displacement

Pre-displacement Experiences of Violence and Loss not Directly

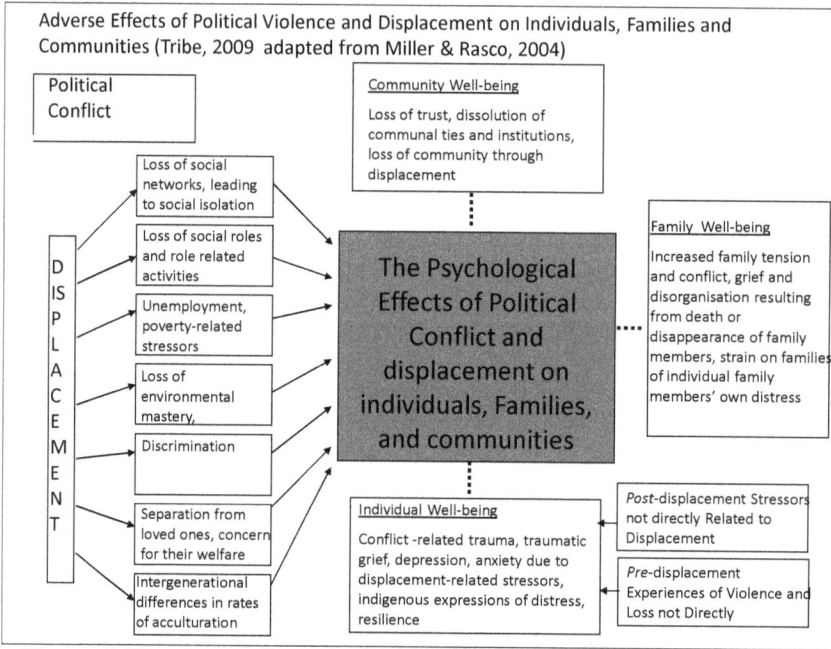

Diagram 1: The adverse effects of political violence and displacement on individuals, families and the communities.

Community Based Rehabilitation

This section of the chapter will briefly describe several community based rehabilitation projects undertaken in Sri Lanka, these are a woman's empowerment project undertaken with groups of women who had been widowed by the war and were resident in refugee camps, a children and carers project, training undertaken forthe Ministry of health and various non governmental organisations (NGOs) and a project we are currently devising which works with military personnel who were left mentally scarred by the 26 year civil war in Sri Lanka. The projects were undertaken in conjunction with two Sri Lankan organisations, the Family Rehabilitation Centre (FRC), the UK Sri Lanka Trauma Group (UKSLTG- www.uksrilankatrauma.org.uk) and our local partner Samuttana.

Women's Empowerment Project (WEP)

This was a Community-Based Rehabilitation project for internally displaced widows living in refugee camps in Sri Lanka as a result of the 26 year civil war which took place there. The WEP included women from the major ethnic groups. Sadly there are approximately 60,000 widows in Sri Lanka whose ages ranged from 18 years of age upwards. The aim of the WEP was to improve the well-being and mental health of displaced Sri Lankan war widows, and our initial needs analysis and experience led us to realize that we needed to be innovative and responsive to the expressed needs of our target population, rather than relying on a traditional health clinic model to offer mental health services to individual women. Gender politics meant that the widows were often marginalised and their difficulties went unrecognised. Drawing on a blend of knowledge andideas from Sri Lankan culture, community resources, and support, psychological theory, group dynamics, plus an empowerment model, the WEP was designed as a brief, supportive intervention focused on building strengths among widows at the small group level. The staff team were almost exclusively Sri Lankan nationals who represented the range of ethnic groups present in the country and therefore had familiarity with the culture, language and traditions of the country."The primary goals of the intervention were to improve ethnic harmony, support and build adaptive coping strategies, and increase socioeconomic knowledge and skills among the women participants. In addition, to helping participants develop their community networks and resources, and to reach as many women as possible, the WEP therefore used a cascade model in which a number of program participants received further training and were employed by local extension offices to provide ongoing support, advice, and advocacy for women in their communities" (Tribe, 2004).

The Women's Empowerment Programme (WEP) was run by the Family Rehabilitation Centre (FRC), a Sri Lankan non-governmental organization whose mission was to work to promote ethnic harmony and community development, and to assist survivors of the war by providing medical and psychological care and increasing socio-economic knowledge.

The Women's Empowerment Programmes were designed to empower Sri Lankan war widows by providing them with access to information, facilitating individual and community-level coping strategies, and drawing on the considerable inner resources of the women themselves. It is a 3-5day groupprogramme. The WEP targeted communities of women, rather than individuals, because offering individual women help might have been viewed as'pathologizing' their difficulties and might have had less impact on precipitating positive change. Although the programme is no longer running as the civil war is over. The WEP ran more than forty times in the majority of Sri Lankan areas where refugee camps were located.

The major components of the programme covered the following areas, though each individual programme would be developed after a needs-analysis conducted in advance with the participants and local organisations. Local resource people are used (as well as members of the staff team) so that they could be strategic in assisting the women and to sensitise them to the specific dilemmas facing the widows.

- Primary health care and first aid (delivered by the local doctor or matron and frequently an ayurvedic or indigenous doctor
- Mental health and well being
- Legal assistance (regarding rights and entitlements delivered by a lawyer form the area)
- Self employment opportunities (conducted by local experts)
- Job finding skills
- Financial affairs

On the last day of the program, women who had previously been through the WEP were invited to return to discuss their experiences of the programme and what they had been able to use from it afterwards. There have been a number of positive outcomes from the WEP which included the establishment of women's groups and several credit unions. Other projects included those making and mending of clothes, mat weaving, catering projects, growing vegetables and herbs, and making paper bags to sell to local stall holders and shops.

Comments from participants included:

"The WEP had assisted her and other participants in using their resources and skills and encouraged them to be brave and courageous so that others would respect what they had to say. We can be role models."

"I came with the hope that I will be able to solve my problems. Now I understand that there are others like myself from other ethnic groups who have undergone the same problems and hardships."

"After my husband was killed, I had no love for life. I was beside myself. . . . After attending the FRC seminar, I began to realize that there were many others affected like me. The kindness, compassion, and training given by FRC helped me to stand on my own two feet. I have learned a lot from these programs and now have the courage to face the future and look after my child."

"We had problems trying to obtain death certificates for our husbands. I am happy to learn from the lawyer who spoke to us how to obtain the death certificates."

"I have decided to form a co-operative society, when I return to the camp, we will start with a small amount. . . . This will enable us to give loans to members for self-employment such as mat weaving or poultry keeping."

A formal evaluation of the WEP was conducted by anindependentinternational organisation, (a summary of these can be located at Tribe, 2004). The evaluators noted in their evaluation "this will be of use to FRC in making more effective the important and opportune task they have dedicated themselves to." With regard to the war widows, the evaluators noted that, "FRC is filling a very important gap by recognizing and targeting this marginalized group. This phenomenon in our country's recent history has yet to reach the public consciousness. As such, FRC's work is certainly both pioneering and opportune."

Children's Activity Project

The children's play activity (Fig 3) is a community rehabilitation project run throughout Sri Lanka between 1992 and 2009. It was started with the objective of working with children and their carers, who had suffered the experience of being exposed to armed conflict, violence, separation, displacement, loss of family members and economic difficulties and were currently living in refugee camps. As the civil war was of 26 years duration, some children and young people have no experience of a life in peace.

It was a multi-level intervention which worked with children, their carers, health and education professionals and community leaders, the programme was set up so that the latter group took over the running of the programme, with some support from our team. The programme was designed using community resources and skills, cultural and psychological knowledge, whilst being based around a more radical model which maximized the considerable internal resources and resilience of the carers, health and education workers, the community and the children themselves. It also drew upon a sharing of the survival strategies, skills and knowledge that the parents, community, education and health workers had used previously. The programme also works directly with the children in providing structured play activities for communities of children.

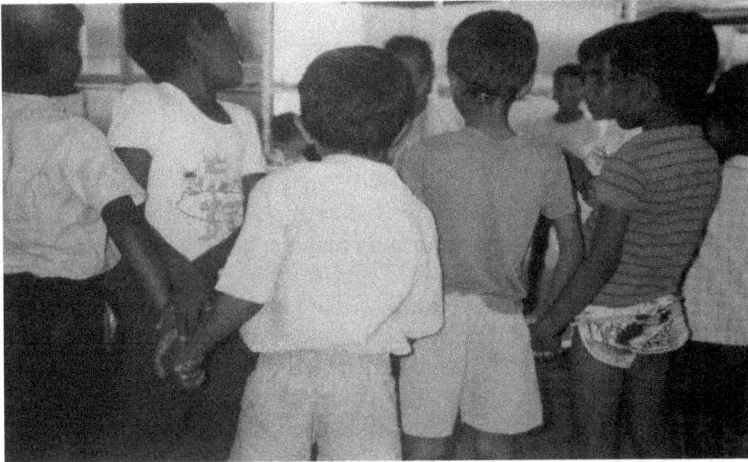

Fig 3. Children's Activity Project

Programme/Intervention Components

The broad objectives of the programme were to:
- identify the psychosocial needs of children exposed to armed conflict and provide interventions to promote healthy growth and development
- enable caretakers, parents, teachers and others interacting with children to identify those most at risk and to feel more confident in themselves and in working with those children to assist them

The programme aims to achieve this by:
- providing a structured environment where the carers' feelings and concerns about their own situation and its effect on their children could be shared and ways of working with this considered;
- developing an intervention programme with local experts and identifying children with emotional difficulties;

- providing knowledge about the needs of children for healthy psychosocial development;
- developing the participants' skills on practical therapeutic play activities, carer or parent involvement and interaction plus other relevant interventions;
- developing skills among the play leaders/carers to conduct training programmes at a basic level using a cascade/waterfall methodology'

We attempted to embed the intervention through using the waterfall or cascade method, in which information and ideas shared or obtained by one group of people within the play activity programme were passed on to another group and thence to a third group of people and so on. This rendered the programme sustainable and assisted with transparency and openness, built capacity and enabled the community of children and carers to own the programmes over time. Systematic monitoring of the programme was undertaken and sustainability constantly reviewed. A full description of this project can be located at Tribe (2004).

Conclusion

This chapter has looked at Cultural Perspectives on Mental Health and Community Based Rehabilitation in Sri Lanka and the importance of considering poor mental health and well-being as containing the potential to be disabling. The importance of considering cultural constructions and context has been emphasised if any rehabilitation projects are to be as helpful as possible to those they are attempting to help. The issue of some western theorists and clinicians assuming that a set of mental health criteria developed in the west can be un-questioningly generalisable world wide is briefly considered. Two examples of community based rehabilitation projects undertaken in Sri Lanka are then described where our team worked with the expressed needs of two specific groups of people (firstly war widows and secondly children and their carers and networks). Both groups of people were living in refugee camps at the time of the interventions, both projects were taken over either entirely or in part and owned by the participants themselves over time, with our team's role changing to one of support and assistance when required thus assisting with sustainability and capacity building. Each project was also formally evaluated each time it ran, with an over all evaluation conducted by an independent organisation. Thus, we were able to constantly refine and develop the programmes over time to try and ensurethey were relevant and useful.

References

Bonanno, G. (2004). Loss, trauma and human resilience: Have we underestimated the human capacity to thrive after extremely aversive events? American Psychologist, 59, 20-28.
Bracken, P. J. & Petty, C. (1999) Rethinking the Trauma Of War. London: Free Association Books.

Byrne, P. (2000) Stigma of mental illness and ways of diminishing it. Advances in Psychiatric Treatment 6: 65-7

Department of Health Information Centre (2011) Attitudes to mental illness www.ic.nhs.uk/pubs/atitudes to mil1 accesses 12.7.12

De Silva, P. (1999) Cultural aspects of Post Traumatic Stress Disorders In Yule, W. Post traumatic Stress Disorders Concepts and Therapy. Chichester: Wiley

Fernando, S. (2010). Mental Health, Race and Culture Basingstoke: Palgrave Macmillan

Goodley, D. (2001) Learning disabilities, the social model of disability and impairment: challenging epistemologies. Disability and Society 16,2,207-31

Human Rights Watch,(2009) www.hrw.org accessed 24.6.2009

Inter-Agency Standing Committee (2007) IASC Guidelines on Mental Health and Psychosocial support in Emergency settings www.who.int/mental_health/emergencies/guidelines_iasc_mental_health _psychosocia ..

McNamee S. & Gergen, K.(1992) (eds) Therapy as Social Construction. London :Sage

Mental Health Foundation, 2012 www.mentalhealth.org.uk accessed 13.7.12

Mind (2012) www.mind.org.uk accessed 12.7.12 ,

Mir, G., Nocon, A., & Ahmad, W., and Jones, L. (2001). Learning difficulties and ethnicity. London: Department of Health.

National Institute for Mental Health www.nimh.nih.gov/ accessed 12.6.12

Office for National Statistic Psychiatric Morbidity report 2001. www.dh.gov.uk / Home / Publications

Reuters, 2009 www.reuters.com/news accessed 12.10.12

Rousseau, C & Measham, T. (2007) Post traumatic suffering as a Source of Transformation : A Clinical perspective in L. J. Kirmayer, R. Lemelson & M. Barad (eds) Understanding

Trauma: Integrating Biological, Clinical and Cultural perspectives. Cambridge: Cambridge University Press p.p.275-93

Royal College of Psychiatrists (2003), www.rcp.org.uk accessed 12.7.12.

Save the Children (2006) www.savethechildren.org.uk/ accessed 20.5.2007

Samarasekera, S.., Amarasekera , N., Davies, M., Siribaddana, S. (2012) The stigma of mental illness in Sri Lanka: the perspectives of community mental health workers. Stigma Research and Action, 2, 2 ,93-99

Somasundaram, D. (2007) Collective trauma in northern Sri Lanka: a qualitative psychosocial-ecological Study. International Journal of Mental Health Systems, 1:5

Somasundaram, D. and Sivayokan, S. (2000) Mental Health in the Tamil Community. Jaffna: Transcultural Psychosocial Organization (sponsored by the World Health Organization).

Summerfield, D. (1999) A critique of seven assumptions behind psychological trauma programmes in war-affected areas. Social Science and Medicine, 48, 1449-1462.

Summerfield, D. (2002) commentary on Tribe, R. Mental Health of refugees and Asylum-seekers. Advances in Psychiatric Treatment, 8, 247

Tribe, R. (2004) A Critical Review of the Evolution of the Children's Play Activity Programmes Run by the Family Rehabilitation Centre (FRC) throughout Sri Lanka. Journal of Refugee Studies,17,1,114-135

Tribe, R. (2007) Health Pluralism - A more appropriate alternative to western models of therapy in the context of the conflict and natural disaster in Sri Lanka? Journal of Refugee Studies, 20.1, 21-36

Chapter 5: Community Based Rehabilitation Disability and Post-coloniality: The Jamaican Context

Patricia Smith

Introduction

In this chapter, I will look at post-colonialism from a historical perspective and current debates which provide the background for understanding disability and cultural identity in the context of a post-colonial setting; works such as Benahabib on post-colonialism which introduces concepts on communitarian values and Nettleford on Jamaican culture and Neo-colonialism which looks at the Jamaican cultural context of post-colonialism, representation, identity and disability. Lastly, I will draw on Nettleford's theory of cultural identity and present the implications of post-colonialism on representation of disability. However, before I present these areas I will give an account of the development of post-colonialism as an area of study. This is based on research which I conducted with the 3D projects, a Community Based Rehabilitation Programme (CBR) in Jamaica. Community Based Rehabilitation was developed as an alternative service programme for people living with disability in developing countries to increase accessibility to rehabilitation and to promote equalization of opportunities for the social integration of disabled people into the community and into society (WHO, 1981). However, one has to be clear that disability is culturally constructed in a situation of social change as in the case of postcolonial Jamaica.

Post-colonialism: A Historical Perspective and Current Debates

According to Nordquist (1998) a search for the history of the colonized led to a series of studies called post-colonialism. Originally, 'post-colonial' had a clearly chronological meaning designating the post-colonial independent period. However since the late 1970s, the term has been used by literary critics to discuss the various cultural effects of colonization (Ashcroft et. al 2000:186). This search for history is exemplified for example in regions such as the Caribbean, which has experienced two of the most extreme forms of exploitation known in human history, slavery and colonialism (Bolles, 1986 & D'Amico-Samuels, 1986). Colonialism, which has been identified as the political conquest of one society by another followed by social domination and cultural change (Lavendah & Schultz, 2000:170) has, as a central theme, the concept of empires and how these empires control and dominate less powerful societies (Said, 1993:44; Lavendah & Schultz, 2000; Nettleford, 1998:96). The dismantling of the colonial control after the Second World War was a unique historical movement that led to the development of post-colonial studies resulting in the reshaping of traditional methods of cultural analysis (Lavendah & Schultz, 2000).

For the most part, post-colonialism has provided a variety of ways to perceive the world and is open to many interpretations. For example, in one interpretation, post-colonialism is often seen as a political strategy (William & Chrisman, 1993:282). According to William and Chrisman (1993:281), post-colonialism and colonial discourse is itself a complex contradictory mode of representation which implicates both the colonizer and the colonized. In post-colonialism, the *object is the imperialist subject, the colonized as formed by the process of imperialism*. Post-colonialism according to Said (1997) produces narratives of progress and development, which were part of the past. However, other authors have said that post-colonialism has the advantage in that it brings to the foreground the politics of opposition and struggle and problemizes the key relationship between centre and periphery, that is, British Imperial rule and the colonized subjects at the periphery (Mishra and Hodge, 1991). In areas of the existence of mankind, the significance of the British Empire as the centre and the colonies such as Jamaica as the periphery is a factor that has an impact on the struggle that people encounter in living with disability, especially poor rural families with disabled children.Post-colonial societies also have their own internal centres and peripheries, their own dominants and 'marginals' which suggests that even within a 'post-colonial' cultural context, there are 'sub-cultures' or different strata operating internally which can affect the wider society (Mukerjee 1998:222).

In another interpretation, post-colonialism is largely about the situation of each individual. Some writers on post-colonialism therefore draw on ideas of identity and gender (Benhabib, 2002; Benhabib, 1991; Bhabha, 1994, Mukerjee, 1998). Other authors have conceptualized post-colonialism by those things which deal with the effects of colonization on cultures and society (Ashcroft et al 2000:186). As such post-colonialism becomes the methodological framework through which such ideological conceptions of gender, ethnicity, identity, class, nationalism, pan-nationalism, cultural awareness, and politics are developed and used in daily living.

Nettleford (1998) and Chevannes (1999) advocate that though physical slavery has ended that there is still a high level of dependency by Jamaica on bigger countries under the banner of post-colonialism. The economic implication of post-colonialism was evident to me as I participated in the life experiences of the participants a study that I conducted with the 3D Projects, a Community Based Rehabilitation programme in Jamaica (Smith, 2006). Discussions of resistance, oppression and representation continue to take place within Jamaican society and it seems that post-colonial theory does not begin at the point of 'independence' as in 'after-colonialism' but that post-colonial theory represents a 'continuous process of imperial suppression and exchanges throughout the diverse range of societies' (Ashcroft et. al. 1995:2). In addition, post-colonialism rejects classification of 'first and third world' and contests the suggestion that post-colonial is synonymous with economically 'under-developed' (Ashcroft et. al. 1995:2).

The present day economic dependency of a country like Jamaica on 'the West' signifies a new type of enslavement known as neo-colonialism which will be described later in this chapter. This has contributed to the economic dependencey that families find themselves in at present. This condition trickles through all levels of Jamaican society, but has its most blatant effects at the lower levels of society where the lack of money to buy the necessities of life in order to provide for the family is a problem (Nettleford, 1998). Post-colonial theory is therefore significant for understanding the Jamaican socio-cultural context of those living with disability. The dynamics of economic dependency have impacted on the lives of disabled children and those living with disability and this is especially so in a post-colonial society.

Post-colonialism features strongly as the tool through which ideas of community, disability, cultural identity, spirituality and the impact this has on the daily lives of individuals in a society. I must however, point out at this stage a key distinction that I will make between the concepts of *post-colonialism* and *post-coloniality*. As Ghandi (1998:8) states, if post-coloniality can be described as the condition troubled by the consequence of a historical dimension, then the value of post-colonialism is seen in part as its ability to elaborate the forgotten memories of this condition. The point I make here is that, in my study of disability, cultural identity and community, I will be looking at the *condition* in which my participants find themselves and how *they* live and express their understanding of it *in their own words*. This is post-coloniality.Post-colonialism then becomes the tool through which this expression is made. I will now present post-colonialism in relation to disability.

Post-colonialism, Disability and Cultural Identity

In discussing cultural identity and health beliefs in a CBR programme, post-colonialist theory gives an understanding of how people view their health and disabilities within their own cultural context following the colonial experience. People living with disability in post-colonial Jamaica were faced with the experience of issues surrounding resistance, suppression, representation, difference and gender. These impacted significantly on the lives of the people that I worked with in my study, particularly in the understanding of 'the self'. To understand 'self' is important in CBR because self is that part of being which does not identify with the resistance, and suppression often associated with disability. Instead, it is the infinite potential to rise above these limitations (whether it be through participation or community involvement) to produce models of functioning which address their own socio-political context.

In all societies, people endeavour to establish a cultural identity that speaks specifically to them. However, in post-colonial societies like Jamaica and the rest of the Commonwealth Caribbean, the question of cultural identity gains high priority alongside political independence and economic self-sufficiency in the process of de-colonization and the struggle against external domination (Nettleford, 1978). How they identify themselves culturally in relation to their disability is, to my mind, a constant process and it is, as Nettleford (1978: xv) states, the combination of economics, politics and culture which determines the timbre of the ideological thrust of many who advocate change. Hooks (1992) defines de-colonisation as a political process and a struggle to define oneself in and beyond the act of resistance to domination. She quotes Hall (1990) from his essay "Cultural Identity and Diaspora" who defines cultural identity as a matter of 'becoming' as well as 'being'. Identity, which looks at the question of personhood belongs to the future as well as to the past and points initially to the self (Gilroy, 1996). I would add that the self is neither in the past or present but is in the ever present. This is key to understanding disability within the context of culture.

Two post colonial theorist informed my work: Seyla Benhabib, a political theorist and Rex Nettleford who was the vice chancellor of the Univerity of the West indies and a prolific writer and theorist. Whilst Benhabib provides an internationalist perspective on post-coloniality and culture, Nettleford gives insight into understanding Jamaican culture which was specific and unique to Jamaica's cultural setting. His work provided a framework for the understanding of culture and politics from the Jamaican perspective, something that aided me greatly in providing a construct in which to debate cultural theory and disability from the perspective of the families. I will talk about how his work addresses issues of identity and self and how this relates to my work with families of disabled children in the climate of neocolonialism/post-colonialism.

Benhabib and Post-colonialism

Benhabib (1992:1) makes clear the expression that one's lived experiences or lived time are 'imbued with symbolic meaning' and in the context of the prevailing forces around us many times there is but a 'dim understanding of the present'. In other words, past experiences influence present experiences and many times the struggles of present experiences dull the memory of past experiences which have brought us to where we are. Her critique of the many "post-isms" such as post structuralism and postmodernism in our cultural lives, led her to conclude that these are "only expressions of a deeply shared sense that certain aspects of our social, symbolic and political universe has been profoundly and most likely irretrievably transformed"(Benhabib 1992:1). I found this quote exceptionally interesting, because during my study, when I spent one year living and moving amongst the families living with disability I shared their experiences. Benhabib's ideas transformed the way in which I was able to observe these expressions. I could see these expressions as though I sat in the front row of a theatre performance, observing and being part of the experiences of the present, which were mingled with experiences of the past. I was in the ever present. Acts of sharing, giving and receiving displayed with one another, in the family and in the community, were acts of transforming their existing reality. This was how they transformed their lives within the socio-cultural context of post-colonialism in Jamaica.

Achebe (1988) suggests that the European ideology of universality make the assumption that everyone is the same. However, Benhabib (1992:3) goes on to argue that in defending the tradition of enlightenment universalism which suggests that there is only one reality or understanding of disability, one has to address the multiplicity of contexts and life situations and take seriously the claims of community and gender. This spoke so clearly to my own work, because when I looked at the lived situations of the families living with disability, I realized just how complex their own situation was and yet how easily they worked together to overcome these complexities. These multiple realities were interdependent and interrelated. What lingers quite deeply in my own mind is how Benhabib (1992:5) recognizes that 'subjects of reason are finite, embodied and fragile creatures and not disembodied or abstract unities'. This goes to the heart of what I purport in this chapter. How those living with disability understand 'self' which is the will to bring forth and achieve their goals of rehabilitation is culturally determined and in the face of post-colonialism it is crucial to the effective delivery of CBR. The self which is consciousness and will (Amen, 1990) is the basis for family and community and is a *'model of the continuity of present and past*. How the families perceive their health in relation to their bodies and how the influences of cultural factors such as economics, religion, spirituality and politics are expressed in a post-colonial cultural setting are necessary for an understanding of what approaches are best suited for this cultural setting.

Further in relation to the generalized and concrete other, Benhabib (1992: 149) makes clear the distinction between the ethical orientations, between justice and rights, as in Kohlberg's (1971) conservative approach to communitarian values and the ethical orientation of care and responsibility in Gilligan's (1982) liberal approach to communitarian values. She supports the view that Gilligan takes when she says that people are immersed in a network of relationships with others and that each other's needs and the mutuality of effort to satisfy them, sustain moral growth and development. This idea has been purported by Etzioni (1998:xi) who advocated that the new communitarians made the question between the individual's rights and social responsibility between autonomy and common good a major concern. This insight appealed to me because the care and responsibility given by the mothers of these disabled children is reflected in the context of the community and in the relationship within the family and the community.

Nettleford: Jamaican Culture and Neo-colonialism

After 'independence' the relationship between former colonies and imperial rulers remained intact, largely in connection with economic links in the form of what has been termed 'Neo-colonialism' (Nettleford, 1993; 1998). This is particularly important for Jamaica, a former colony, and the implications for this in relation to disability are far-reaching. One such effect is what scholars have called cultural imperialism (Said, 1972: xxviii, Lavenda & Schultz 2000:172), a situation whereby the ideas of and practices of one culture are imposed upon other cultures. This is important because western ideas and understanding of disability and family relationships may differ from other cultures.

It suggests that although ex-colonial countries had gained 'technical' independence, the ex-colonial powers and newly emerged superpowers continued a decisive role through international monetary bodies, multinational corporations, cartels and a variety of educational and cultural institutions (Nettleford, 1978). Needless to say, the effect of neo-colonialism is also reflected in the health sector and has impacted on issues of disability particularly for those who are poor and do not have access to institutional resources either because of distance or lack of money. To explain this I present this scenario. Under neo-colonialism, the government may need to seek financial aid from the World Bank, but in order to meet the target to qualify, government spending has to be cut. Government does not see disability issues as a priority, hence adequate funding may not be available to, or it may be removed from, government sectors including social services, education, transportation and health services. People living with disability and their families in rural communities would therefore find it difficult to get appropriate transportation to access these health institutions and this becomes an additional cultural imperative as a result of dependency on 'developed' countries. Because of lack of national resources, spending on social services is cut in order for the government to meet its own needs.

Jamaica gained 'independence' from British rule on the 6th August 1962. Since then Jamaica has been economically dependent on 'developed' countries in most aspects of its economy, even though the International Monetary Fund (IMF) has described Jamaica in the 1960s as an "upper middle class income" country with a free market and dominant private sector (Leavitt, 1992: 52 & 53). However, in present day Jamaica, the legacy of the colonial era and the continuation of post-coloniality present real problems in Jamaican society, often reflected in economic underdevelopment and recession, poverty, unemployment, crime and environmental degradation (Nettleford, 1998). In addition, post-coloniality has led to a high level of migration of families abroad, mainly to Canada, the United States of America and Great Britain, resulting in breakdown and changes in family structure (Statin, 1991: Nettleford 1998:). This has resulted in remittance families, who depend on financial support from family members abroad.

Nettleford (1978; 1993) suggests that confusion over the matter of identity is rife. In addition, he speaks clearly of the transculturation process whereby people of African ancestry, which includes most of rural Jamaica, have been Europeanized and have, to a large extent, taken on the ideals and values of their past colonial masters. This was significant to my research on disability in Jamaica, because in Jamaica, there were issues surrounding identity. Being able to understand the cultural implications of one's identity in relation to their disability became a mammoth task in the delivery of CBR. This is a major cause for concern, because in the delivery of CBR, (its ethos being the use of local resources in rehabilitation WHO, 2001; WCPT News, 1998: 4; Thomas & Thomas 2002:83), a people who look outside of themselves, through 'European' eyes may underestimate their own creativity and ingenuity in developing the means and resources needed to address their needs and the needs of their disabled children. Nettleford alludes to this creative capacity of Jamaicans (Nettleford, 1998).

Nettleford also addresses the issues of cultural identity and cultural resistance, Caribbean history and the quest for knowledge, the battle for space, the creative imagination and intellect of Jamaicans. This has implications for how disability is perceived and handled in the face of neo-colonialism. Poor families in rural Jamaica, who cannot afford to buy toiletries or ambulatory aids for their children because of the effects of the devaluation of the dollar, make the harsh reality of CBR in Jamaica a challenge for Jamaicans who use the service. Nettleford (1993:51) says this explicitly when he states that in Jamaica's pursuit for cultural identity and the essential unity of an individual, the Caribbean development and the shaping of new societies in the form of social living shifts the power base from colonialism to independence. This gives rise to an artistic creation, which has long been a phenomenon in Caribbean and Jamaican society. This creativity was very apparent in the families that I worked with. During my research in Jamaica (Smith, 2006), I observed the way in which families and CRWs made corner chairs, crutches, walking frames and toys for the children out of the material resources around them. This was an act of both ingenuity and creative impulse. What was most compelling was the pride with which this was done and the joy expressed by those who used them. Most Jamaicans are therefore challenged to fall back on their own inner reserves of historical experience and cultural dynamics in order to exist on their own terms which is partly what cultural identity is all about (Nettleford, 1993:57).

Another issue Nettleford (1998) raises with regards to the effects of post-colonialism in Jamaica is the contextualizing of class, colour, and race specific to Jamaica; (this is an area not analyzed through Benhabib's work). There are several strata of skin colour in Jamaica, which is closely related to class structure in Jamaica (Nettleford, 1998: 34; Spencer-Strachan, 1992:42-43). In this class structure, the elite were often white, or 'brown skinned' and were at the higher social strata whereas the poorer, often rural, Jamaicans were 'black skinned'. The notion of class structure is one that Spivak (1990) defines as artificial and economic and 'the economic agency or interest is impersonal because it is systematic and heterogeneous'. Spivak (1990) says further that in the postcolonial context, the description of 'black' or 'colour' loses its persuasive significance. The effect of this is that for the poorer black-skinned Jamaican, psychologically, he or she may not possess as strong a racial memory of great cultural achievement as his European, Chinese and White compatriots (Nettleford, 1998:35). This has implications on the imperceptible nature of the 'self' and how the colonial past has impacted on the post-colonial present which in turn has implications on disability and CBR in Jamaica. For a child with a disability, a poor family living in rural Jamaica often has to contend with perceptions of identity in relation to their 'persons' and their child's disability, which is often seen in a negative light rather than in relation to the self and the infinite potential to achieve a positive outcome to their goals of rehabilitation. Furthermore, as Nettleford (1998:35) goes on to say, the African of all the groups which came to the New World, came as individuals and not as part of their language group. Hence they were unable to maintain group identity through great religious activity and other recognized customs. The obvious answer for the black Jamaican was to submerge his or her racial consciousness in the wider and greater aspiration to acquire education and other means of making himself or herself economically viable. Cultural identity and health beliefs also have implications for representation, identity and disability which I will discuss next.

Representation, Identity and Disability in the Post-colonial Context

Representation can speak to the political process and Hooks (1992) defines de-colonisation as a political process and a struggle to define oneself in and beyond the act of resistance to domination. This political process is addressed in the context of CBR where CBR is seen as a process concerned with social change in terms of attitudes, knowledge and skills (AHRTAG, 1993). This social transformation enhances the quality of life and activities of daily living (ADLs) within the community by way of aids and equipments thereby enabling people with disabilities (PWD) to participate in local life (AHRTAG, 1993; Abberly, 1987; Barnes, 1992).

For a person living with disability in a Jamaican socio-cultural context, this dynamic representation of present and past is important because the goals of physiotherapy intervention in CBR will be determined by what they, the recipient, want to 'become' and how they want to be represented or visually seen. How people define themselves within the context of their health or disability is therefore linked to their culture. It is agreed in the literature that the term culture is one that is difficult to define and has evolved in meaning over the years (Baldwin et.al. 2004:3; Smith, 2001:1; Kroeber & Kluckhon, 1963:77). However, amidst the myriad of definitions or meanings given to the term 'culture', the one that I will use in this chapter is defined as the entire way of life, activities and customs of a people, group or society (Smith, 2001:2). I will use the understanding of culture, not as a constraining factor but culture as the ability to enable action (Smith, 2001:5).

Cultural identity and people's ideas about health may dictate the attitude and approach that recipients may have towards CBR. Although studies have been conducted addressing aspects of cultural and social attitudes in CBR (Thorburn, 1998; Bischoff et. al. 1996) more research needs to be carried out to address these issues in more detail.

Implications of Cultural Representation and Disability in the Jamaican Context

I will now introduce some issues surrounding the cultural representation of disability and speak about the implications of this in the Jamaican cultural setting. In my work in Jamaica, self-image speaks a lot about one's own status in the community. For the family that has a disabled child, this may raise in the minds of the parents and other members of the community questions of self-worth or self-actualisation and self-blame and not least the physical capabilities both for the child and the parents. In the Jamaican media, disability may still be seen in a negative light even though attempts have been made to change this image through television programmes such as the Jamaican Information Services and through the National Policy on Children. Some of these issues were highlighted in an interview that I carried out in 2002 with a cabinet minister in the Jamaican Government who himself has a physical disability. He spoke about his own commitment to raising the profile of disabled people in society by creating positive representation of disabled people to the public. He suggested that this had been done mostly with respect to people who are blind. Physically and mentally disabled children had yet to be given the public attention needed to create the necessary positive image. This lack of attention was due mainly to economic reasons, but there was also, he believed, a need for a change in the national culture of thinking about disabilities as a whole in order to enhance this positive image.

The implication of representation in my own work was that families who already saw themselves in a negative light by virtue of their disabled child may have been less willing to participate in a CBR programme of rehabilitation in a culture where people with disability are not valued. This may have implications for the child. Families may feel that 'all is lost' and that there isn't much to gain from such interventions. Generally within Jamaican culture and media, very little is done to modify the negative representation of people living with disability.

Understanding the whole notion of representation in disability guided me in my own approach to working with those with disabilities and their families. For my own work, the challenge was for me to allow the participants through their own acts of symbolism (words and imagery) to express how they perceived their personhood (Gertz, 1993:61). Spivak (1990) makes the distinction between two types of representation: representation as 'speaking for' as in politics and representation and re-presentation as in the art of philosophy. Spivak (1990) then says that the theoretician does not represent (speak for) the oppressed group. This I found useful in my own approach to relating to the disabled and the family. An example of this is when during a period of play activities with one disabled child and their parents, the children may draw pictures of themselves in the park. Secondly, in talking casually with parents I may ask them to talk about their own thoughts on what their child's disability means to them. For many, it was a question of their child being dependent on them for the basic things in life, the consequence being the parent's own sacrifice of their own aspirations in order to meet the needs of their child. This was important, because as Katrak (1989: 163) states,

> "Language is a culture, especially the transformation of rhetorical and discursive tools available through a colonial(ist) education system; and one expression of cultural tradition (among others like film, popular culture festival) is through language"

Health as part of a cultural tradition fits into this category and therefore language used for representation is significant to CBR and my study. I say this because from my observation, disability can have either a negative or positive effect on self-image and level of participation in CBR.

I feel, however, that the way health and disability have been represented (for example in the media) may have an impact on how someone interprets and gives meaning to their understanding of disability within their own culture, a notion that others have noted (Hall, 1997; Shakespeare, 1994). Shakespeare (1994) discusses the prejudices underlying the representation of disabled people in for example, the media, where they are often viewed as objects rather than subjects.

He makes reference to imagery in the form of cartoons, television and photography where disabled people are seen as passive and incapable, thus creating a negative image. He also speaks about the part that charities play in creating "demeaning images of disabled people" thereby engendering pity and sympathy in 'normal' people. These images may well influence families' perception of themselves and their disabled children in such a way that it may question their status or self-esteem in the community.

Post-coloniality & Disability in the Jamaican Context

In addressing cultural identity and health beliefs in a Jamaican context, one cannot do this in isolation from the impact of the post-colonial experience on the understanding of one's view of health, especially in relation to disability. According to Mallory (1993:5), the primary historical factor that informs one's beliefs about disability in non-western societies is the effect of colonial occupation beginning in the 17th century and reaching a peak in the 19th century. This time period was marked by the exploitation of man and natural resources by European cultural ideals and values leading to unequal distribution of resources between western and non-western societies. This unequal distribution of resources was correlated with the incidence of disability in that less resources where available for those living with disability (Mallory (1993:5). As such, disabled persons often define their problems not in terms of individual impairment but in terms of social oppression (French, 1997:65). Furthermore, Uprety (1997) establishes a link between disability and post-coloniality when he says that commonalities have been identified in these two areas with respect to behavioural patterns of the oppressed disabled and the oppressed person in a post-colonial society.

This kind of oppression in Jamaican society is echoed in a study by Chevannes & Levy (1996: 45) which depicts the emergence of the colonial past into the 'post-colonial' present and the effect on families living with disability. It was found that historically, the residents of an old inner city urban community turned spontaneously to the past to give meaning, through the continuities and the differences to current happenings and conditions. For example, they would refer to the 'good old days' when people use to 'live good' and often associated with this was the music of the time such as 'rock steady' music by the Skattelites and Count Ossie. They would recount with pride the commercial self sufficiency in the form of bakeries, hardware stores, Community Enterprise Organizations and a rich 'corner life' fed by 'corner discussions', 'dancehall' and a 'wonderful theatre'. The cost of living was more tolerable and certainly not the oppressive burden it is today. There was a sense of freedom such that in spite of not having all the material things, you could walk the streets freely without fear of being molested. This kind of image conjures up a real understanding of the sense of community spirit that existed in the early 1960s and the kind of environment that a disabled child and family would find themselves in."The emergence of post-colonialism and its effect of poverty, crime and unemployment impact on the environment in which people with disabilities (PWD) live and their *ability* to realise their full potential of self because their construction of the past and present are interrelated" (Gilroy, 1996:52). This provides a kind of explanatory self-reflective model of what people living with disability want to do and why they want to do what they want to do.

As I reflected on these sentiments, it occurred to me that disability had within it its own social pressures, because in addition to dealing with the physical limitations of disability, those living with disability had to deal with the limitations of self actualization and living up to society's standards. A person or family experiencing this oppression would quite likely have to come to terms with their own feelings of self worth and self identity as part of a group as they endeavoured to participate fully in society. French (1997:87) suggests that research in the area of disability should therefore struggle against social oppression and remove barriers to full participation. This oppression is especially poignant in a post-colonial era where there is a connection between post-colonial theory, culture theory and social responsibility.

It appears to me that, in a community setting, a theory of CBR should be based on social responsibility, which takes into account the post-colonial experience. Social responsibility may become a vehicle through which CBR can be expressed as a practical process within its own cultural context (AHRTAG, 1993). A practical example that I use is how CBR's approach to the use of toys in the rehabilitation process is culturally related to the child. This idea is echoed by Katrak (1982) in her essay on the 'de-colonising of culture towards a theory for post-colonial women's text'. She saw the concept of social responsibility as the basis for any theorising on post-colonial literature. She suggests that social responsibility can then become a "strategy to consider certain integral dialectic relationships between theory and practice" (1982:95). However, when one considers theory and practice, one sees that Imperialism, which is the practice and attitudes of a dominating metropolitan centre ruling a distant territory, is in itself still present. Imperialism did not suddenly pass when decolonization had set in motion the demantling of classical empires (Said, 1993:34) and in the Jamaican society, legacies of the past Imperial rule still stand as a reminder of that period (Nettleford, 1978:32).

Within a discourse on disability and self-identity, the retention of traditional practices and health beliefs in rural Jamaican society might be one of cultural resistance. Nyman & Stotesury (1999:19) describe cultural resistance as refusing to be controlled, and in this perspective, cultural resistance should 'manifest in social process in multiple events involving immediate practical issues, but also less tangible agendas of resisting perceptible dominant forces' (op.cit :19). For example, the integration of traditional African religious practices and western religious beliefs produces many cultural forms of worship and expressions of spirituality. Nettleford (1993:99) refers to this when he says:

> Dance preserves its own force through integrated links with religion and worship with forbidden but persistent Gods, divination rituals and the configuration of the nether world beyond the master's law. This finds its expression in forms such as Kumina, Zion, revivalism, Etu, Gerreh, Tambu, Pukkumania and Rastafarianism

The significance is that when a disabled child and family comes into a religious context which integrates African and western religious beliefs, there is an amalgamation of physical illness and spiritual illness that is viewed as a continuum. For people living with disability and especially for physiotherapists working within a CBR programme, understanding this connection may be important for the effective outcome of rehabilitation.

Post-coloniality and Religious Beliefs

In this section I consider the impact of the missionary movement that accompanied colonization. According to Mallory (1993:7) the missionary movement brought with it not only the Christian ideals it professed, but also traits of paternalism, chauvinism and ideological conversion as a requisite for salvation. Out of this, a paternalistic relationship developed whereby the benefactors provided educational institutions and those benefitting were not educated in their own language or culture. I find this interesting from the viewpoint that in my work as a community physiotherapist, for some, disability is often linked with ideas of reliance or dependence, while for others disability represented a resolution to rise above paternalism and oppressive treatment. Some of these residual attitudes are reinforced as post-colonial countries such as Jamaica continue to adopt Western policies and practices with respect to the treatment of people with disabilities. As such, the legacy of the missionary movement is the reliance on voluntary non-governmental services to marginalized groups rather than the use of more formal, state operated and funded services (Mallory, 1993).

In physiotherapy practice in a post-colonial society, understanding the relationship between post-coloniality and religious beliefs is therefore very relevant. The way that people in a post-colonial era have been presented with ideas and understanding of religion and healing and how one responds to a disability have come out of western ideologies of health and religious beliefs (Mallory, 1993). Jamaican people have developed their own patterns of survival and resistance which is often depicted in the language used to express their experience and view of health, disability and religion. There can be marked national and cultural differences in perceptions of and beliefs about the nature and cause of illnesses.

I reiterate Noorderhaven's (1999) suggestion that care needs to be taken when working in other cultures, so that practitioners should not necessarily treat the patient how they (the practitioner) want them to be treated, but instead how *they* the (recipients) want to be treated. This is important because according to Ristock & Pennell (1996) empowerment as an approach to community based research means thinking consciously about power relations, cultural context and social action. The phrase 'research as empowerment' conveys the idea that research itself can be a lived process of empowerment when it encompasses both a critical analysis of power and reconstructs power so that the latter can be used in a constructive manner Noorderhaven's (1999).

Conclusion

In this chapter I introduced ideas around the historical development of post-colonialism, disability, politics and cultural identities which are relevant to the discourse of health issues, particularly physiotherapy practice in a community-based setting. I presented elements of Benhabib's theory on communitarian values and the understanding of self (Amen, 1980). I also presented Nettleford's (1990) theory on cultural identity and the effects of neo-colonialism on 'self' and 'identity' in the Jamaican cultural setting. I then introduced the concept of representation and how the person living with disability has been constructed in the post-colonial context, making special reference to the Jamaican setting. I concluded with a look at post-colonialism and religion and the impact of the missionary movement during colonization.

References

Abberley, P (1987) The Concept of Oppression and the Development of a Social Theory of Disability. *Disability, Handicap and Society*, 2 (1) 5-19.

AHRTAG (1993) *Annual Report and Accounts of Spastics Societyof Tamil Nadu, India.*

Amen Ra Un Nefer (1990) *Metu Neter Vol 1 The Great Oracle of Tehuti and the Egyptian System of Spiritual Cultivation. Khamitic Publications*

Ashcroft, B; Griffiths, G; Tiffin, H (2000) *Post-Colonial Studies: The Key Concepts.* Routeledge.

Ashcroft, B.; Griffiths,G.; Tiffin, H. (1994) *The Post-Colonial Studies Reader.* Routledge, London & NewYork.

Baldwin, E.; Longhurst, B.; Smith, G.; McCraken,S.; Ogborn, M (2004) *Introducing Cultural Studies.* (Pearson) Prentice Hall.

Banks, M. E (2004) Disability in the Family: A Life Span Perspective. *Cultural Diversity and Ethnic Minority Psychology.* 9:367-384.

Barnes, C. (1992) *Disabling Imaging and the Media.* Halifax: The British Council of Organizations of Disabled People and Ryburn Publishing Limited.

Benhabib, S (2002) *The Claims of Culture, Equality and Diversity in the Global Era.* Princeton, NY Oxford.

Benhabib, S (1992) *Situating the Self: Gender, Community and Postmodernism in Contemporary Ethics.* Polity Press.

Bhabha, H (1994) *The Location of Culture.* New York. Routlegde Press.

Bischoff, R., Thorburn, M. J., Reitmaier, P (1996) *Neighbourhood support to families with a disabled child: Observations on a Coping Strategy of Care-Givers in a Jamaican Community-Based Rehabilitation Programme. Child: Care Health andDevelopment,* 22,397-410

Chevannes, B. (1999) *Lecture Series: What We Sow and What We Reap: Problems in the Cultivation of Male Identity in Jamaica.* Pub Grace Kennedy Foundation lecture.

Chevannes, B; Levy, H (1996) *They Cry 'Respect': Urban Violence and Poverty in Jamaica.* Published by the Centre for Population, Community and Social Change, Department of Sociology and Social Work, University of the West Indies.

French, S. (1997) *Physiotherapy: A Psychosocial Approach*, 2nd Edition. Butterworth-Heinemann, Oxford.

Geertz, G (1993) *The Interpretation of Cultures.* Fontana Press.

Ghandi, L (1998) Postcolonial Theory, a Critical Introduction. Allen & Unwin.

Gilroy, P. (1996). *Cultural Studies and Communication: British Cultural Studies and the Pitfalls of Identity*. Arnold Press.

Hall, S. (1990) Cultural Identity and Diaspora in *Identity: Community, Culture Difference*, Ed. J Rutherford. London. Lawrence & Wishart.

Hooks, B. (1992) *Black Looks: Race and Representation*. Turnaround Publishing.

Katrak, K (1989) *Decolonizing Culture: Towards a Theory for Post-colonial Women's Texts*. MFS 35 (1) 157-79.

Kroeber, A. L.; Kluckhonn, N (1963) *Culture: A Critical Review of Concepts and Definitions*. Vintage Books.

Lavenda, R. H.; Schultz, E. A. (2000) *Core Concepts in Cultural Anthropology*. Mayfield Publishing Co.

Leavitt, R. L. (1992) *Disability and Rehabilitation in Rural Jamaica: An Ethnographic Study*. Associated University Press Inc.

Mallory, B. L. (1993) Changing Beliefs About Disability in Developing Countries: Historical Factors and Sociocultural Variables. IEEIR Monograph No. 53 *Traditional and Changing Views of Disability in Developing Societies: Causes, Consequences, Cautions*. University of New Hampshire Press

Mukerjee, A (1998) *Postcolonialism, My Living*. Toronto.

Nettleford, R. M. (1978) *Caribbean Cultural Identity: The Case of Jamaica: An Essay in Cultural dynamics*. Publishers, Institute of Jamaica.

Nettleford, R (1993) *Inward Stretch, Outward Reach: A Voice from the Caribbean*. Macmillan Caribbean.

Nettleford, R. M (1998) *Mirror, Mirror: Identity, Race and Protest in Jamaica*. Kingston Publishers Limited.

Noorderhaven, N. G. (1999) Intercultural Difference: Consequences for the Physical Therapy Profession. *Physiotherapy*, 85, 504-510.

Nordquist, J. (1998) Social Theory: A Bibliography. No: 50 – Post-colonial Theory.

Rickstock J.P; Pennell J. (1996) *Community Research as Empowerment – Feminist Links, Postmodern Interruptions*. Oxford University Press.

Said, E. (1993) *Culture and Imperialism*. Chattoo & Windus, Vintage.

Said, E (1997) *Cultural Readings of Imperialism*. Lawrence and Wishart London.

Shakespeare, T (1994) Cultural Representation of Disabled People: dustbins for disavowal? *Disability and Society*, 3, 283- 299.

Smith, P (2001) *Cultural Theory: An Introduction*. Blackwell Publishing.

Smith, S (1996) Ethnographic Enquiry in Physiotherapy Research: The Role of Self in Qualitative Research. *Physiotherapy*, 82, 349-52.

Smith, P (2006): A Cultural Approach to Community Based Rehabilitation and the Implications for Physiotherapy Practice: Unpublished PhD Thesis. University of East London.

Spencer-Strachan, L (1992) *Confronting the Color Crisis in the Afrikan Disaspora: Emphasis Jamaica*. Afrikan World Infosystem, New York.

Spivak, G (1990) *The Post-colonial Critic: Interviews, Strategies, Dialogues*. Ed Sarah Harasym, New York, Routledge

Statin (1991) Statistical Institute of Jamaica

Thomas, M; Thomas, M. J. (2002) A Discussion on Some Controversies in Community Based Rehabilitation*Pacific Disability Rehabilitation Journal*, 13, (1)

Thorburn M. J (1998) AttitudesTowards Childhood Disability in Three Areas in Jamaica. *Asia Pacific Disability Rehabilitation Journal*, 9, (1) 20-24.

Uprety, S. M (1997) *Disability and Postcoloniality in Salman Rushdie's Midnights Children and Third World Novels chapter 21* in Davis, L. J. (1997) The Disabilities Studies Reader. Routledge.

Williams, P; Chrisman, L (1993) Colonial Discourse and Postcolonial Theory: A Reader. *Chapter 4. Can the Subaltern Speak, Spivak, Gayatri Chakravorty.* Harverst Wheatshift.

WCPT *Therapy News* (1998) Issues 2 pg. 4

World Health Organizations (1981) *Disability, Prevention and Rehabilitation. Report of the WHO Expert Committee on Disability Prevention and Rehabilitation. Geneva, Switzerland. World Health Organization.*

World Health Organizations (2001) ICF: *International Classification of Functioning, Disability and Health.* Geneva.

Chapter 6: Cultural Competence and Disability: A Lifelong Journey to Cultural Proficiency, Part I

Ronnie Leavitt

Introduction to Cultural Competence

Does the duck that quacks the loudest get shot or does the squeaky wheel get the grease? The answer might depend upon how you view the world - what assumptions you make about the nature of reality and what cultural value system you reflect. Today, with the recognition that we increasingly live in a multicultural world with a wide range of people with disabilities, health professionals and life ways, it becomes apparent that there is no one correct answer.

The need for cultural competence presumes that diversity is a given and positive. Within the health care system, a greater understanding of how or why people think or behave in a particular manner can lead to increasing positive outcomes. Therefore, there can be improved patient outcomes with regard to functional ability and/ or quality of life, as well as improved levels of professional and personal satisfaction for the health care professionals who would feel more competent at their job.

The field of cross-cultural health has begun to flourish and the idea that cultural competence is desirable and necessary has become more widely accepted. Demographic transitions, substantial disparities in health outcomes among ethnic, disability, and cultural groups, and the moral imperative to treat individuals by a gold standard, have led to the development of regulatory and accreditation standards regarding cultural competence. Ruth Purtilo has called for cultural competence to be a non-negotiable skill, tested as rigorously as competence in any bio-medical or other field of study (Purtilo 2000).

This chapter hopes to introduce some of the key facts about cultural competence and to open the way to a better understanding of its relationship to disability. It discusses what cultural competence is and what cultural competence is not and how the health professional can become more equipped in dealing with issues of cultural differences. Lastly it looks at how the theoretical models of cultural competence can assist in this process.

Cultural Competence: What is it?

There is an increasing body of literature on definitions and theoretical models describing cultural competence. Arguably, the most relevant and thorough definition of cultural competence, is that developed by Cross et al (1989).

> *Cultural competence* is a set of behaviours, attitudes, and policies that come together in a continuum to enable a health care system, agency, or individual rehabilitation practitioner to function effectively in trans-cultural interactions. In practice, cultural competence acknowledges and incorporates—at all levels—the importance of culture, the assessment of cross-cultural relations, the need to be aware of the dynamics resulting from cultural differences, the expansion of cultural knowledge, and the adaptation of services to meet culturally unique needs (Cross et al 1989).

Cultural competence is an essential element in making an effective and efficient examination, evaluation, diagnosis, prognosis, and intervention possible. Developing rapport, collecting and synthesizing patient data, recognizing personal functional concerns, and developing the plan of care for a particular patient requires cultural competence. The practitioner who sees a wide range of functional impairments is expected to meet the needs of a patient within the context of that patient, the patient's family and community, and the broader cultural setting. By reviewing information on some of the unique characteristics associated with the patient, one may gain insight and adapt the patient-practitioner interaction and the rehabilitation services provided to create the best plan of care possible.

Understanding the concept of culture is the key to understanding cultural competence. The concept of culture has been defined in dozens of ways going back to the 19th Century. Tylor (1871/1958) defined culture as "that complex and whole which includes knowledge, belief, art, morals, law, custom, and any other capabilities and habits acquired by man [sic] as a member of society" (p.1). Lynch and Hanson (1998) describe *culture* as the framework that guides and bounds life practices.

People do not biologically inherit a culture, they learn it. People may share cultural tendencies and pass these tendencies to the next generation. However, cultural frameworks are never rigid, and they are constantly evolving. Many factors - such as ethnic identification, socioeconomic status, migration history, gender, age, religion, and physical capabilities - have a profound effect on a person's way of life. A person's culture is closely interrelated to value systems, health beliefs and behaviors, and communication styles. Based on these variables, people may be members of several *subcultures* which are smaller, but in some ways distinct, units within a larger culture (Loveland 1999). Cultures may have many similarities and differences among them: One's culture is not inherently better or worse than any other.

In every interaction, the practitioner will need to consider, minimally, four specific cultural milieus. The practitioner's own culture, the patient's culture, the culture of the specific profession, and the culture of the health care system/organization in which the interaction is taking place should all be considered in the practitioner-patient relationship. To be culturally competent a practitioner must (Cross et al 1989, Leavitt 1999):

1. *Acknowledge the immense influence of culture.* This is the most important concept, to explore. It is essential to understand that all people are immersed in their own culture—with its associated beliefs, attitudes, and behaviors—which guides their personal and professional interactions. However, human nature is such that everyone tends to be *ethnocentric*, believing that their own cultural way of life is the norm and the standard by which all others are judged. What we forget is that the next person, who may be from another culture, also may be ethnocentric. Thus, the relevance of this self-awareness (or lack of it) is especially critical when health professionals work with patients who come from different cultures. I do not believe that one can properly succeed at steps two through four if this step is passed over.

2. *Assess cross-cultural relations and be vigilant concerning the dynamics that result from cultural differences.* With cross-cultural interaction comes the possibility that the other person's intentions and actions may be misjudged. Each party brings a specific set of experiences and personal and communication styles to an interaction. Clinicians must be vigilant to minimize misperception, misinterpretation, and misjudgement through improved communication and thoughtfulness. With more insight into the patient's or client's perspective—and fewer stereotypes—the ability to develop a mutually advantageous relationship is bound to be enhanced.

3. *Expand our cultural knowledge and incorporate this knowledge into our everyday practice.* If we assume that health care professionals can work effectively with people from other backgrounds, increased knowledge about the patient or client's socio-cultural context can only improve the relationship. Clinicians must seek out socio-cultural information that will then help them appropriately modify an interview or history—what questions to ask and how to ask them—and modify interventions based on a person's cultural reality. Health professionals should ask patients questions about their culture and lifestyle and indicate their willingness to learn about that culture. In that way, each party in the interaction can understand the wish to both give and receive information. Clinicians must be aware of the ethnographic makeup of the local community and the relevant beliefs and behaviours of their patients and the patients' families.

4. *Adapt to diversity.* Professionals need to develop culturally sensitive examination and intervention practices that allow a patient to be comfortable during the visit. The health care environment should be adapted to create a better fit between the needs of the people requiring services and the needs of the clinicians and staff.

It is important to remember that cultural competence is *NOT*:

1. abandoning your own culture and becoming a member of another culture by taking on all of the attitudes, values, and behaviors of that culture.
2. asking our patients to abandon their culture and take on the attitudes, values, and behaviors of your culture.
3. learning everything about all cultures and subcultures. This is impossible, and unnecessary.
4. assuming one person speaks for an entire group of people.
5. assuming that a person's health concern is attributable only to socio-cultural factors and that it is not necessary to examine the patient for physiological pathology.
6. cultural relativism:it is unrealistic to presume that one will not make judgments about other cultural practices. Few would deny that there can be cultural practices that are deemed by some to be detrimental to others with regard to health.
7. being "politically correct".
8. a quick fix. Although some relatively small actions such as changing the décor of a waiting area, or hiring a person of colour, can make a difference in a client's comfort level, this alone is not cultural competence. Rather, the life long journey of achieving cultural proficiency requires changes that go deeper - a systematic appraisal and attempt to meet the requirements discussed above.

Cross et al (1989) described 6 stages along a continuum of cultural competence ranging from cultural destructiveness to cultural proficiency (Table 1). In my view and based on my 45 years of experience in physical therapy and public health, most health professionals and health care institutions are moving from stage 3 (cultural blindness) to stage 4 (cultural pre-competence). In cultural blindness, clinicians and health care institutions assume that they are unbiased. However, this assumption is based on an incorrect belief that all people are the same. In this stage, facility policies and practices do not recognize the need for culturally specific approaches to solve problems. Cultural pre-competence lies toward the more positive end of the continuum. In this stage, clinicians recognize weaknesses in the health care delivery system or in their personal cultural knowledge base, and they explore alternatives. They are also committed to responding appropriately to cultural differences. Cultural competence is stage 5, and the last stage is cultural proficiency where there is recognition for the need to conduct research, disseminate the results, and develop new approaches that might increase culturally competent practice.

Table 1. The Continuum of Cultural Competence

Stage	Name	Definition
1	Cultural destructiveness	People are treated in a dehumanizing manner and are denied services on purpose.
2	Cultural incapacity	Health care systems are unable to effectively work with patients from other cultures; bias, paternalism, and stereotypes exist.
3	Cultural blindness	Presumption is that all people are the same and that no bias exists; policies and practice do not recognize the need for culturally specific approaches to problem solving; services are ethnocentric and encourage assimilation; patients are blamed for their problems.
4	Cultural pre-competence	Health care system is committed to using appropriate response to cultural differences; weaknesses are acknowledged and alternatives are sought.
5	Cultural competence	Cultural differences are accepted and respected; continuous expansion of cultural knowledge and resources and continuous adaptation of services occur; continuous self-assessment about culture and vigilance toward the dynamics of cultural differences exists.
6	Cultural proficiency	Cultural differences are highly regarded; the need for research on cultural differences and the development of new approaches to enhance culturally competent practice is recognized.

Theoretical Models of Cultural Competence

Theorists and health practitioners have developed models and/or approaches to foster cultural proficiency. Some of the more widely accepted and utilized are described here. Reviewing these models (and assessment tools should allow the reader to more fully understand the robust nature of cultural competence. All the models imply that cultural competence is a never-ending, always evolving, non-linear process that will continue to challenge us. All of these are similar, yet distinct enough to warrant recognition.

Arguably, the model used most often after Cross et al (1989) is that described by Josephina Camphina-Bacote (2003). Campinha-Bacote, (2003) defines "cultural competence" as "the process in which the healthcare provider continuously strives to achieve the ability to effectively work within the cultural context of a client, individual, family, or community" (Campinha-Bacote, 2003, p.54). Her model has five essential constructs that are interdependent and necessary to reach cultural competence.

1. Having cultural desire ("the motivation of the healthcare professional to 'want to' engage in the process of becoming culturally competent;" (2003 p.15)is described first. It presumes the ability to sacrifice one's prejudice and biases toward those who are different and "includes a passion and commitment to be open and flexible with others; a respect for differences, yet a commitment to build upon similarities; a willingness to learn from clients and others as cultural informants; and a sense of humility" (2003 p.16).
2. Having cultural awareness ("cultural sensitivity" is often the term used), requires considerable self-examination regarding one's own biases and the recognition of one's own cultural beliefs, values, and behaviors. Becoming culturally aware requires both cognitive and self-awareness, learning about others, and integrating a range of approaches and world views.
3. Increasing cultural knowledge requires seeking information about different groups in order to understand the theoretical and conceptual frameworks of others. This can cover a range of domains but the general worldview and value system, health-related beliefs and behaviors, disease incidence and prevalence, and treatment efficacy are especially important.
4. Developing cultural skills necessitates the ability to collect culturally relevant data in a culturally appropriate way in order to develop a culturally relevant treatment plan.
5. Having a cultural encounter is the exposure to people from different cultures with an opportunity to help them achieve shared goals.

Campinha-Bacote (2007) has also described a cultural competence continuum.that moves from unconscious incompetence (having a "cultural blind spot" or assuming there are no differences in culture between the professional and client) to conscious incompetence (recognizing one's lack of knowledge) to conscious competence (learning about other peoples' cultures, verifying generalizations, and adapting interventions to be culturally appropriate) to unconscious competence (spontaneously providing culturally relevant care for diverse patients). At this later stage, the process is natural and comfortable (Campinha-Bacote 2003).

Yet another framework is Borkan and Neher's (1991) Developmental Model of Ethnosensitivitythat assesses the healthcare workers' ability to grasp cultural issues by describing a continuum from ethnocentrism to ethnosensitivity. The practitioner moves from fear (mistrust) to denial (cultural blindness, overgeneralization) to superiority (negative stereotyping) to minimization (reductionism) to relativism (acceptance) to empathy (pluralism) to a final stage of being ethnosensitive or the ability to appreciate values and behaviours within the context of specific cultural norms and to apply this ability to healthcare practice.

Anthropologist Milton Bennett (1993) has suggested a continuum that begins with avoidance and progresses to integration as a final stage. The first three stages are considered ethnocentric and the last three ethnorelative:

> Denial / Avoidance - a person denies cultural differences or is unaware that others do not share a similar world view

> Defense / Protection – although a person acknowledges the existence of differences, these are considered threatening to one's sense of self. Defense mechanisms must be employed such as denigration of others and believing in one's own superiority.

> Minimization – an individual trivializes the cultural differences that exist and focuses on presumed similarities (i.e. person x is just like me) in an effort to emphasize humanity as a unified group.

> Acceptance – cultural worldviews are recognized and accepted but the individual is more focused on behaviors as opposed to values.

> Adaptation – individuals improve skills to interact and communicate with people from other cultures.

> Integration – people value a range of cultures and work toward conscious evaluation of alternative behavior and values. These individuals try to integrate aspects of their own culture and those from other cultures into clinical practice.

More recently, Schim et al (2007), apply a puzzle metaphor to understand culturally congruent care. The puzzle represents a non-linear and inter-connected visual tying the constructs together. The model is still evolving but the four basic constructs for the health care provider are cultural diversity (a fact of life), cultural awareness (the cognitive construct), cultural sensitivity (the affective or attitudinal construct), and cultural competence (the behavioural construct). The client layer of the model is equally important. It recognizes individuals, families, and communities.

Conclusion

This chapter has introduced some of the key facts about cultural competency and its relationship to disability. Cultural competency embraces the idea of cross-cultural health and health and rehabilitation professionals are just beginning to explore the issues associated with disability when viewed from a broader social perspective. Cultural competence is as important as clinical competence. It is our professional moral imperative to embrace cultural diversity and move towards cultural proficiency as we develop the most appropriate service models and public policy to enhance the lives of all people with disability.

References

Bennett, M. J., (1993). Towards ethnorelativism: A developmental model of intercultural sensitivity. In R. M. Paige (ed.) Education for the intercultural experience. Yarmouth, ME: Intercultural Press

Borkan, J. & Neher, J (1991)*A developmental model of ethnicity in family practice training. Family Medicine,* 23 (3), 212-217.

Campinha-Bacote J (2007) The Process of Cultural Competence in the Delivery of Healthcare Services: The Journey Continues, 5th edition

Cross TL, Bazron BJ, Dennis KW, Isaacs MR (1989) *Towards a Culturally Competent System of Care: A Monograph on Effective Services for Minority Children Who Are Severely Emotionally Disturbed.* Vol 1. Washington, DC: Georgetown University, National Technical Assistance Center for Children's Mental Health.

Leavitt RL, ed. (1999) *Cross-Cultural Rehabilitation: An International Perspective.* London, England: WB Saunders Co..

Loveland C. The concept of culture. (1999) In: Leavitt RL, ed. *Cross-Cultural Rehabilitation: An International Perspective.* London, England: WB Saunders Co :15–24.

Purtilo RB (2000) Thirty-First Mary McMillan Lecture: A time to harvest, a time to sow: ethics for a shifting landscape. *Phys Ther.* 80:1112-1119.

Schim S., Doorenbos, A., Benkert R., Miller J (2007) *Culturally Congruent Care: Putting the Puzzle Together . J of Transcultural Nursing;* Vol. 18, No. 2 pp 103-110.

Tylor E. B. (1958) Primitive culture. New York: Torchbooks. (Original work published in 1871)

Section II: The Culture of Professional Practice

Chapter 7: Cultural Imperatives within Community Based Physiotherapy: Narratives from Families Living with Disability

Patricia Smith

Introduction

This chapter will look at how cultural imperatives are manifested in Community Based Rehabilitation programmes (CBR). I will use narratives from families who were living with children with disabilities. According to Leavitt (2010) Community Based Rehabilitation (CBR) has its roots in the provision of rehabilitation services for people who have limited access to rehabilitation services. In the case of many developing countries such as Jamaica, there may be many reasons for this e.g., cost, lack of resources, environmental barriers to name a few. The philosophical principles that underpin Community Based Rehabilitation are equal access, equal opportunity and integration into mainstream community life at all levels (Leavitt, 2010). As such the success of CBR programmes in the Jamaican cultural context depended greatly on how belief systems influence people and dictate their activities.

In a qualitative study which I conducted in St. Thomas, a rural community in Jamaica (Smith, 2006), I spent one year carrying out interviews and participant observation of eight families that lived with children with varying degrees of physical disability. Community life was central to family life. Cultural imperatives such as building relationships in a spirit of community, sharing resources, and community capacity building were necessary for successful rehabilitation of the child and the family. These cultural imperatives guided people's behaviour and thinking. They were necessary for successful rehabilitation.

Below are excerpts from my study with some quotes that speak directly to these imperatives.

The Spirit of Community

The Jamaican political and social context has been strife with warfare resistance, unemployment and a social class divide. However, in spite of the tensions of political warfare, my study found that there was still evidence of caring and sharing within the community between neighbours and friends. It was clear that there was no division between community and family. In many cases, the family was the community and the community was the family. One author (Some, 1997) talks of the community as 'the spirit', the guiding light where the 'tribe' comes together to fulfill a specific purpose and to take care of one another. This network of support and sharing is again seen in the case of Akita, one of the participants in my study. Akita was eight years old and lived with her mother Fumni in a tenement 'yard' with her three other sisters and a small baby brother. The tenement yard, that small, open area in the yard that was bordered by three wooden houses and a small church served as the communal meeting spot. Everything took place there. All doors opened to this area where the children played, where washing and cooking were done, women combed each other's hair and general conversations took place. Hairdressing is an informal occupation among women done free and sometimes paid where working for oneself is preferred (Chevannes 1996).

This was a family yard, historically handed down from earlier generations (Fumni's grandparents). That was the space where people come to share spirit, meaning that space where they can talk about the things that bothered them. In this setting there didn't seem to be a distinction between the private and the public domain. Everything happened in one space, which would probably not be the case in the western tradition. As Benhabib (1992:5) points out, one of the chief contributions of feminist thought to political theory in the western tradition is to have questioned the line dividing the public from the private. She argued that the 'privacy' of the private sphere which has always included the relationships of the male head of the household to his spouse and children, has been an opaque glass rendering women and their traditional spheres of activity invisible and inaudible Benhabib (1992:5). Women and the activities to which they have been historically confined such as child-rearing, house-keeping, tending to the sick and the elderly (and in the case of this study even the disabled child) have been placed until very recently beyond the pale of justice. The norms of freedom, equality and reciprocity stood at the household door (Benhabib, 1992:13).

My own research identified that the poorer communities usually have a common area where everyone knows each other, the exchange of support the women gave to each other was a natural development. For example, whenever mother Fumni was not around and she had to go out for any reason, Akita, the disabled child, was taken care of by Sheryl, one of the other tenants. She was like a second mother to Akita. This bought to my mind what Karenga (1997) describes as communitarian values in which he describes traditional African philosophical thinking, which places a stress on communitarian values. This philosophy, a tradition he states, carries with it an understanding of the person and the community as 'one', a conception which underpins communitarian values (Karenga, 1977). He goes on further to state that there are three basic assumptions underlying these values. Firstly the person is never isolated from the community, in others words, the person and the community are one. The community defines the person. Secondly, the view of personhood is one where personhood is seen as a process of becoming and not simply a state of being. Hence, there are successive stages of integration of the person into the community through the rituals of rites of passage, which mark important life cycles such as birth, naming, adulthood, marriage and death. Karenga (1997) goes on to say that real and truly respected personhood must be achieved after a long process of 'social and ritual transformation' in which a person attains the moral intellectual and social values seen as truly definitive of personhood. In this long process the community plays a vital role of catalyst and prescriber of norms.

Other authors have also spoken about the importance of communitarian values (Mbiti, 1975, Etzioni, 2004, 1998; Arthur, 2000). Mbiti (1975) sees the person and the community as a symbiotic investment in each others' wellbeing, happiness and development. He states that it is only in the consciousness of others that one becomes conscious of one's own duties privileges and responsibilities towards oneself and towards other people. This notion has been described by Etzioni (2004:14) as the balance between individuals and groups, rights and responsibilities and among the institutions of state, market and civil society. Etzioni (2004:13) advocates that this communitarian perspective recognizes both individual human dignity and the social dimension of human existence. Maintaining institutions in society which promote respect for others and respect for oneself, skills of self-governance and service to others are features of a communitarian perspective (Etzioni, 2004:13).

Hence, whatever happens to the community happens to the individual, and whatever happens to the individual, happens to the community. This communitarian value system is not restrictive or oppressive as might be perceived in the context of a European value system but respects the interdependence and reciprocity of the person and the community a notion that Etzioni (2004:21) has described as social justice, and Amen (2003) explains as Maat (Law). Furthermore communitarian values encourages the development of a 'responsive community' in which the basic needs of individuals in a community are met (Etzioni, 2004:15).

For the family living with disability and the community into which this child is born, the understanding of self, capabilities of speech and action, and expectations for that child relate directly to the value placed on that child and the value placed on the relationship of the community to that child.

Community Capacity Building

I recall how this sense of 'community' and what may be seen as an assumed network support system became apparent to me in the case of Cherry and Chrissy. Cherry lived in a one room concrete house with her husband, twenty-year-old son and her three-year-old child Chrissy who had cerebral palsy. Chrissy was a 'floppy' child meaning that she had very low tone in all her muscle groups and was unable to carry out any voluntary movements and as such she functioned at the level of a three-month old baby. She was unable to sit up independently, roll or do other activities. She was heavily dependent on her mother Cherry. Cherry stayed at home to look after her 'baby' and operated a lunch and catering business from her home where she cooked meals which she sold to members of the community. As Nettleford (1978) points out, people have to use their skills with flexibility and ingenuity in order to create employment for themselves, a notion which SHIA (2002:8 & 9) refers to as ownership of CBR and community capacity building. Cherry provided a service to her small communal area. The community in that sense was that cluster of small homes where people gathered and shared information. Several things were happening in that 'little community'. Young men gathered under a tree playing dominoes and would come to Cherry's kitchen to buy food at lunch time, then would go back under the tree to continue their game. People were sharing information such as telling each other what was on the menu from Cherry's kitchen (which served as her home kitchen and business kitchen). This ability to earn from home was what Cherry needed to be able to do to have the money to buy medication for her disabled child and to have the taxi fare to take her to the doctor when necessary. Her ability to care for her child depended on her ability to generate an income. The emotional support, the financial support, the presence of others around were all important to provide the physical aspects of looking after a disabled child. In her own frustrations she would 'cry out' for support yet she seemed to have a determination that in spite of all this she felt it her duty and responsibility to take care of her child. She spoke a lot about an inner strength that she drew on that empowered her in coping with her child. Yet she would sometimes talk about the guilt she felt about having a disabled child and the effects that this had on her relationship with her husband as he often had to work long hours.

Children in the community came to order their soup from Cherry's kitchen. It was obvious that the soup was well received by everyone in the community and the word got around that Miss Cherry's soup 'tastes good' and therefore everyone came to order. Cherry began to realise that she didn't cook enough soup as it was running out and she had to save some for herself, her husband and for Chrissy. She said that she didn't know the soup would have gone so well and that it looked like she may have to do more, but couldn't be bothered now as she was tired and it is going to take too much time and effort now. She decided to do some plain rice and chicken instead for anyone else who come to buy lunch. She went inside and she lay Chrissy on the bed. Immediately she began attending to her cooking business, selling to people as they came to buy. I looked at Chrissy in the bed who was now quite curled up in her marked extensor pattern, fussing and crying quite a bit. Cherry then talked about someone who asked her if she would have anymore children. She said to me that she told them, no, she was too old for that now and she have Chrissy who needs her attention. If she has anymore now that means she wouldn't have enough time for Chrissy and at this stage in her life she can't bother with that now. It would mean more time to care for another child and she would not have the time. Chrissy is enough work at present. Her frustrations she was experiencing with her caring for Chrissy and the strain on her relationship with her husband was evident in her words:

> "sometimes mi feel like dis is some kind a punishment. But me know seh God will help mi. Mi husband seh a my fault mek di baby come disable."

> "Sometimes I feel as if this is some kind of punishment. But I know God will help me. My husband says it is my fault that the child is disabled."

In spite of this Cherry often talked about the support that she got from those in her community. She always expressed how everyone in her community had common problems that everyone shared which each other in a caring manner. She felt relationships were built when people had to work together in one-ness. This was evident to me when one day I saw a little girl from next door to Cherry come running into the room to volunteer to 'watch over' Chrissy when Cherry had to go out and needed someone to stay with the child.

This kind of unspoken built-in system of support was at the level of assumption and appeared to be part of the fabric of that small community. It became clear to me at that point in time that what then becomes the 'community' is the little girl who comes from next door to stay and play with Cherry's disabled child. She is providing a service to Cherry within a natural context. The community may be that church sister who passes by to 'offer a word of prayer' to talk about how Cherry is coping and to encourage her.

I recall another participant, mother Tika who had a similar experience to this. She lived in a one room board house in the hills of St. Thomas and had an eleven year old disabled child Runika who was one of twins. She was born severely brain damaged. Tika farmed the plot of leased land and reared chickens from home so that she could look after her child. She sometimes relied on her mother-in-law who lived on the plot of land next door to keep an eye on her child if she had to go 'to town'. Sometimes she had friends who would pass by her house on the way to their house further up the hill and they would come in for a friendly chat and play with the child.

> "Miss P, mi might not have no whole heap a money but yuh si me, me jus wan know seh she have food fi eat, she clean and she can shi dung and watch di rest a we. Mi no tink seh nothing can do fi har now. Mi just a gwann do di exercise when mi can manage sometime mi tek har down a di riva or mek har get some sea water fi help di limb dem. Miss P mi glad seh yuh deh 'bout fi help mi."

> "Miss P, I might not have a lot of money, but as long as she is clean has food and can sit and watch the rest of us in the family, that is fine with me. I don't think she will get better, but I still continue the exercise when I am able. Sometime I take her to the river or the sea to exercise her legs. MissP I am glad you are here to help me."

In a family living with disability, coping is more acute as the needs or demands of a child with a disability are greater. Models of CBR that bodies such as WHO (1989) give to developing countries implicitly have within them Eurocentric assumptions of what they see 'the community' to be. This concept is based on western ideals and ideology. The assumptions of community that underpin WHO models of CBR are often inconsistent with what is experienced as 'the community' for developing countries and what the reality of that community means to them.

Universal Moral Respect and the Concrete Other

I recall very clearly how for one mother, lack of money had affected her life in relation to her disabled child. Her name is Delores and her 11-year-old daughter named Asante was a paraplegic from birth. Delores was self-employed and ran her own business, which involved 'buying and selling' in the market. This is a common phenomenon in Jamaican society and as Chevannes & Levy (1996) state, employment in Jamaica often requires flexibility and ingenuity. They lived in a two-room part-concrete and part-wooden house with a zinc roof on a large plot of land in the rural parish of St. Thomas. Their neighbours lived in similar homes and were scattered along the hillside at varying distances from each other. Delores had nine children, five of whom were living with her; the other four were adults living elsewhere. The children all had the same father except for the last child and they ranged in age from five to eleven years, Asante being the eldest. Asante spent a lot of her time sitting out in an old wheelchair either at the side of the house or under a shady tree in the yard. She was always smiling happily and wanted to participate in whatever the rest of the family was doing. She grew attached to me and always wanted to play games or have me read to her or draw pictures. She had good upper limb strength and function but was unable to move her legs, which had become very contracted due to increased muscle tone.

The whole experience of how a mother could endeavour to care for a disabled child and the impact on that care brought home to me a real awareness of how very positively creative this mother was in earning a living and providing for herself and her children. This brings to my mind what Benhabib (1992) speaks about when she says that self identity is constituted by a narrative unity which integrates what 'I can do, have done and will accomplish with what you expect of me' (Benhabib, 1992:5). What was most striking to me however, was what Delores was able to achieve in the ever present (Amen 1980). It seemed to me that Delores had to identify with who she was and what was expected of her in the Jamaican post-colonial context. She had to provide for her 'children' first and foremost, in a society which was also trying to come to terms with its own identity as a 'nation' (Nettleford, 1978).

This dilemma of an 'individual identity' and a 'national identity' in the Jamaican post-colonial context seems almost like a reflection of one on the other in that what happens nationally affects the individual. This idea seems similar to what Benhabib (1992:10) talks about when she says that the 'relationship of the generalized to the concrete can be seen as a model of continuum' in that a concrete individual is part of a general community or nation and not separate from it. In the first place she says, there is the universalistic commitment to the consideration that every man or woman is worthy of universal moral respect (Benhabib, 1992:10). The standpoint of the concrete other by contrast is implicit in those relationships in which we are always immersed in the world.Part of Community Based Rehabilitation is based on this moral relationship of respect for 'otherness'. Hence, Delores, as an individual worthy of respect, grappling with the decisions of how to care for her disabled child, is also as part of a family as spouse, mother. She has to find the means to know how to reason from the standpoint of the concrete other as stated by Benhabib (1992:10). Hence for Delores, acting within this ethical relationship demands her being able to think from the standpoint of her disabled child. To stand in such an ethical relationship means that as concrete individuals we know what is expected of us by virtue of the kind of social bonds which tie us to one another (Benhabib, 1992: 10) as could be reflected in the case of Delores and Asante.

I was very aware of the tensions and conflict between the decisions that mothers like Delores has to make in being at home to holistically 'enable' Asante to become functionally rehabilitated in the normal home environment, as opposed to an institution. This decision, based on economic reasons, was a serious issue for the participants of this study. There would be implications of earning and living for Delores if she was to abandon her income earning capacity so that she could look after her disabled child. Similarly, the consequences would be far reaching in relation to the impact on that child in not having the advantage of rehabilitation within the normal home environment; to become 'alienated' from her own family if placed in an institution.

As I spent time with this family, the 'community' of love and sharing that they expressed with each other was so clear. Love was expressed in the little things such as helping to feed or dress Asante, getting a glass of juice for her, or the children helping their mother to keep the house clean. All of these showed how each member of that family identified 'the other' in themselves. When they looked at their brother or sister, they saw themselves; when they looked at their mother, they saw themselves. What I found even more compelling was that it was not just the action of fetching a glass of water but the manner in which it was done which seemed to say 'I care about you'. From a rehabilitation point of view not only were the family seemingly confirming Asante's identity as a person by their actions towards her but they were also inspiring her to want to 'do for her self' by reciprocating. This clearly exemplifies what Benhabib (1992:159) talks about when she says that 'our relation to the other is governed by *equity* and *complementary reciprocity*: each is entitled to expect and to assume from the other, forms of behaviour through which the other feels recognized and confirmed as a concrete individual being with specific needs, talents and capabilities. They are norms of friendship, love and care (Benhabib, 1992).

Conclusion

This chapter looked at the narratives of families living with disabilities in a rural Jamaican community and how community capacity building and the spirit of community engendered feelings of oneness and unity amongst the families and the communities in which they lived. This was against the background of resistance, strife and warfare which speak to the dichotomy within post-colonial Jamaica. Moral respect and the notions of being responsible for each other within families and communities promoted creativity and ingenuity in providing community based rehabilitation for children living with a disability.

References

Amen Ra Un Nefer (2003) Maat, the 11 Laws of God. Kamit Publicaions Incorporated.

Amen Ra Un Nefer (1990) *Metu Neter Vol 1 The Great Oracle of Tehuti and the Egyptian System of Spiritual Cultivation. Khamitic Publications*

Arthur, J (2000) Schools and Community: The Communitarian Agenda in Education. Falmer Press.

Benhabib, S (1992) *Situating the Self: Gender, Community and Postmodernism in Contemporary Ethics*. Polity Press.

Chevannes, B; Levy, H (1996) *They Cry 'Respect': Urban Violence and Poverty in Jamaica*. Published by the Centre for Population, Community and Social Change, Department of Sociology and Social Work, University of the West Indies.

Etzioni A (1998) The Essential Communitarian Reader. Rowman and Littlefield.

Etzioni, A (2004) From Empire to Community: A New Approach to International Relations. Palgrave MacMillan

Etzioni, A (2004) The Communtarian Reader: Beyond the Essentials. Rowman & Littlefield Publishers Inc.

Karenga, M (1977) *Kwanzaa: A Celebration of Family, Community and Culture*. University of Sankore Press, Los Angeles.

Leavitt (2010) Cultural Competence: A Lifelong Journey to Cultural Proficiency. Slack Books.

Mbiti, J. S (1975) Introduction to African Religion. Heinemann.

Nettleford, R. M. (1978) *Caribbean Cultural Identity: The Case of Jamaica: An Essay in Cultural dynamics*. Publishers, Institute of Jamaica.

Some, S. E (1997) The Spirit of Intimacy: Ancient African Teachings in the Way of Relationships. Newleaf.

Smith, P (2006) A Cultural Approach to Community Based Rehabilitation and It Implications for Physiotherapy Practice. Unpublished PhD thesis. University of East London.

SHIA/WHO (2002) *Community Based Rehabilitation as we have experienced it. Voices of Persons with Disabilities. Part 1.*

SHIA/WHO (2002) *Community Based Rehabilitation as we have experienced it. Voices of Persons with Disabilities. Part 2.*

WHO (1998) *Community Based Rehabilitation: A Collaborative Document Developed by World Confederation Of Physical Therapist Africa Region with the participation of 2 African Countries*. Uganda.

Chapter 8: "It's Always in My Backpack: Living with Multiple Sclerosis—Conny's story

Fiona McGowan

Conny, aged 52, lives in Wedde, a small rural village in the province of Groningen in the North Netherlands. She has known her husband, Dick for 32 years. Married for 24 years, they have two adult daughters. On the 31st December 2010 her neurologist confirmed that she had MS. The following excerpts are taken from conversations with Conny, recorded during visits with Erlinde, her occupational therapist. Though Conny is fluent in English, Erlinde was able to assist – where necessary – with translation.

The Diagnosis: Offering Opportunities

Since around the time I was 25, I had several minor illnesses. I had problems with my eyes, my left eye did not focus and sometimes everything seemed double. I could not read a paper or a book. I also had difficulty with walking and my legs did not do what I wanted them to do. I found it hard to keep my balance when I was walking. I also had problems with the sensitivity in my hands and feet and sometimes in other parts of my body. I was always thinking and doubting myself because the doctor said that there is nothing wrong with you. It didn't give me the room to look beyond…….it was holding me back from enjoying life and looking properly at life because I was always thinking I am not functioning like I used to or like I was supposed to at my age. So when I got the diagnosis [of MS] it gave me that room and it opened up possibilities. Well,at school I had learned a lot about MS so I know what It is and I know it is not hopeful …or it could be not hopeful…but I was very relieved when I got the diagnosis because I didn't have to doubt myself anymore. It gave me the opportunity to say '*OK now I know, so this is what it is, it is MS*' Now I accept that there are several things I cannot do any more or will not be able to do in the future. But there are also many things I can do and I have to look everyday at what is possible and what gives me, what I call the 'flow'. It can be just little moments, but these give me more room to enjoy things, even just little things.

Since the diagnosis, yes my life has changed, I am less active. In the last 2 years it went very fast the downwards way. Two years ago I still played games, I played tennis matches but now, well this is not possible any more. It went very fast but now there is a sort of steadiness, gives a kind of easier way. During this time, the last two years, it was as if every day was a surprise, how the day would be and what the day would bring. Now it is about five days that it goes well, then a day or two not so good, but then that is like in normal life for everyone, they have days that are good and then you have those 'other' days when things don't go so well.

Work and Leisure: Opening a Box of Possibilities

I used to ride my bike to work, it is about 16 kilometers to Stadskanal and sometimes I would go to Veendam which is 20 kms. I used to work 3 days a week. If I wasn't on my bike then I would be on the crosstrainer for 45 minutes several days a week. I used to play tennis twice a week for a few hours. My husband and I used to walk especially when the girls were teenagers. We would always walk after dinner so we could talk to each other without them hearing everything. On Sunday morning we would walk before we drank coffee. I always felt like I have to do it but once I had a walk around 6km but then I had to be picked up by car. I couldn't walk any further and then I was not able to walk freely, I had to hold my husband, I get a feeling.....well, it is like being drunk. But I have to keep doing it, I thought if I have to just sit on the couch then it can only get worse.

I worked in psychiatry; I worked with patients with chronic psychiatric illnesses. I worked with them for recovery and rehabilitation. I didn't do diagnosis, but I look at the possibilities for them and with them. I would talk to them, and say well, you have your diagnosis but you aren't your diagnosis. You are a human being with your own wishes and you have your own power. So how do you live with your illness but also with your wishes and your power and how can you now have some good things and some fun in your life. This is now what I do for myself and it has helped me very, very much. I have been doing this for the last six years and now, well I see how every patient has their own story and every patient has their own possibilities. It sort of opens a box in your head and helps you to look at things in different ways. It helped me to see what is possible in my life, how to view things differently and also think about the different aspects of life.

What I also want to add is that I have learnt that you have to ask for help. Everyone wants to do things themselves but I have learnt to ask for help. There are things I cannot do anymore, the things I like to do. I like to sew but now I can't draw the pattern. Now I have someone who draws the pattern for me and I have a neighbor who helps me to see if it fits properly and she also helps me with the cutting. Then I can use the sewing machine. I ask for help and now I can sew again. It is very slow but I love it. It was a difficult process. I was a bit afraid of what would happen if it didn't work. I had to think, '*do I want to put so much energy into this, is it worth it?*' It took me a year to make a start. If it doesn't work then I will not be happy, then I have to move on and start with something else. I knew something had to switch in my head, but I couldn't do it, it took me time and it was a process to make that step.

Relationships: Choices and Connections

My MS. It is a part of me. I cannot deny it. You can try to say it isn't there but then I could not live my life like I do now. If you deny it, then you are fighting it and I think that when you are fighting you are losing. You have to accept it and live with it. It is as if in life you are a hiker with a backpack and there are several things in your backpack. And for me, MS is one of those things that is always in my backpack. You have some things in your bag that you are carrying that are always there. It is one of those things. There are a few things that you always carry. There is no choice. In the beginning it took up a lot of space in the rucksack but it is getting less and less. Now there is more space for other things and it is not the only thing in there that I think is important. I also think humour is a thing that is always there. Other things you make a choice about, you decide to take with you or you don't. You may think that, '*well, today I take this thing with me*'' or '*today I take it out'*. But with the MS, I cannot ever take it out. It goes with me.

It is difficult, yes, to live with lower energy and I miss the things I always did with my husband, walking and the biking. It was a sort of connection between us, now we have to look for another connection. It was a connection we didn't have to even think about, it was just there. My husband is out walking now…on his own …. we cannot do it together. Well, we can only when I am with the wheel chair but it is not the same, it is very different. And it is so beautiful around here, the small paths… the nature, normally we could walk from out from the back garden and go by the water, but not now, I can't do that.

Now our daughters are 23 and 21. They are not at home, they live in Groningen. The family, they are supportive and well, they make fun of me a lot. Yes, they make fun of me. Partly as a way of coping and I think it is a good thing. Because then we don't deny it and so it can give an opening to talk about it without making it too heavy. If you cannot make fun of it and you cannot talk about it then you miss a kind of connection.

My friends, well, a lot of my friends live in other parts of the country and they stay friends from when I lived there. Now they cannot see me so much. It gives another view in their minds about what I can do or what I cannot do. Last time a friend called me and I said '*I don't speak too long as I am very tired and I have had a few bad days and, you know, been a little bit ill.*' Then very soon I got mails from six other friends…"*oh we heard it is not good with you ....you are ill ...oh dear*". They think as they cannot see me they interpret things differently. With one girlfriend I really have to watch my words. Also I have to do it with my mum. She lives 250km away. So I always say it is going pretty well and then tell her a little bit more when I am with her when she can see me.

Mobility: Independence, Boots and Ankles

I can still do a lot but I have to plan things more. Before I could hop from here to there but then on the way I could think '*oh I will go here'*, but I cannot do that anymore. Now have to I plan to do that one thing and really nothing else. And well, that is how it is now. I have to organize very much. Before I used to do everything. It was like I was working in my own circus. Very busy and well, now it is less and I am much more organized andsometimes I think'*I can do this or that today*'but then I don't. I think *'yes I will go there today*'but then I have to put the wheel chair in the car, then I need to get the car back by 6 for Dick, then I see there is rain coming, then I think of what I need to take.......and then it is too much work. If I am here in the house or garden I can still walk around. I can drive and I can park in front of the shops if I am just getting one or two things and there are not so many people around. But when I walk it is harder, I have to concentrate on the walking and when there are other people around and in the way it is very difficult. I can walk about half a kilometer and then I go 'drunk'.

Well I have a wheelchair with electric wheels which are helping, a bit like an electric bike, really easy, but not always, it is harder when you go uphill or when it is a bit steep. Well, I kind of like it. I got lessons from Erlinde how to do the steps and I liked it, I thought *'yes I can go now'*. It gives me more freedom with the wheel chair. Before I had to be pushed by someone, now I can go by myself. Erlinde said 'I could do it like this' and well, off I went and did it. It has given me more independence. Well it is also something that goes on in your head, it gives you the feeling of independence. I don't always go outdoors with the wheelchair, but the fact that I can and I know I can, it gives me a feeling of freedom in my head.

It is easy around here, there are not so many people around here. It is quiet, well on Queens' Day* you don't go to the city. I was in Amsterdam a few months ago and well I thought I went crazy. All I saw was boots, boots and people were walking fast and slow and walking in front of me. I really had to watch where I was riding and all the time looking at boots, I had the feeling that I was going to scream. And nobody was looking at me. You have the feeling that people will look to see where they are going but they are only looking out for themselves. It was very difficult and I didn't like it at all. In Groningen it is OK, because there are not so many people on the streets.

People can be negative, they can have that attitude to you, like in the shops some people want to cross before you. I also had sometimes that I was looking for clothes and sometimes somebody just pushes your wheel chair away. I have had it now about three times and I thought *'What? What is this?'* Yes, some people are very narrow minded that they want to do their own things and they don't want to have you in their path. But then I ride into the ankles of some people if they want to get past meand then they look and see it is me in the wheelchair and I think,*'yes, look at me, I did that!'*

From the hospital I had rehabilitation. That was fine but my wheelchair, the wheels don't work well anymore. I am waiting for my own electric wheels for 3 weeks now. The system here doesn't work so well. You have to phone many, many times and keep on with it. The communication doesn't work so well. But well, I do have a fantastic bike with three wheels. I am lying back in my bike. I use it a lot, I am very happy with it. It was provided from the Gementee*. I try to bike every day, it makes me very happy.

Learning To Live My Life My Way

I am responsible for my care. In terms of checking I go to the neurologist and physiotherapist. And if I need Erlinde I can call. That's it but I think it is up to me. I am responsible and I have to check and when things are not going so well I talk with physio or the doctor. I ask *'what can I do or what should I do?'* I think I am already a positive person but the diagnosis helped me not to have expectations that I could not reach. Before that I always thought if I trained a lot I could reach my goals. And now I think that, well, I cannot reach it so now I don't have to work so much for it. It is very important I think that once you have the diagnosis you have to listen to yourself. But I think that is true for everyone on this earth, not only me, to listen for yourself. To live your own life. You must look to yourself, not to other people, thinking that they do this and they do that. Then I too, that I am supposed to do this or that. In a way it is a little bit easier now I have MS because I don't have to say *'no I don't do that because I don't want to'*. I can use my MS a little bit as an excuse. It helps me to take myself more seriously. Maybe it is part of the process in life.

When he was 80 my father taught me something. He said that when you get to the stage when you know everything there is to know about life and about yourself, when you know all that, then it is time to leave. Until that time you are still learning. So the MS helps me a little bit to keep learning more. About life and about me. And I know that I am not supposed to die yet.

Reflective Comments

Yes, this is my story and reading through this was confrontational. After the interviews I had a few days when it is all in my head and I thought *'oh I didn't say this and I didn't say that'. I* realised there are some very simple things I cannot do anymore. But after the talks I realised I didn't think of it as it was not in my focus any more. I am beyond it. But by talking about it, it bought all the things back again. So for a few nights it kept me busy. Some things I forgot as they are not part of my normal life anymore. I am a few steps ahead in the process, it kept me busy thinking and well, I realise it is not necessary to add all those things – they are not a part of my life anymore, it is in the past, I am beyondit, I realise there are some things I cannot do anymore. A normal person could do it, I didn't even think to say something about it, as it is not in my life anymore. It is a part of the process in accepting several things in your life and sometimes it is good to be shaken up a bit then things settle down again in the right place.

I am not really so different as a person from three years ago. Last week we went out on the tandem and my husband and I sat on a bench, beautiful sky, so blue and white clouds. We looked at the birds in the sky and behind us, little birds are whistling. I sat there and I thought,' I am just happy'. We are here on the bike, together on the bench, sitting and looking. And I am happy. *'Yes'*, he said, *'me too'*. Then it doesn't matter if you have MS or not, we were together sitting, enjoying the moment, then afterwards we go on the bike back home. And that is life. You can make it difficult – or it can be very simple.

Glossary

*Queen's Day – National holiday to mark the Queen's birthday.
*Gementee – municipality (http://gemeente.groningen.nl/english)

Further reading:

Barnes, C & Mercer, G (2010) *Exploring Disability* (2nd ed). Cambridge: Polity
      Press

Kinebanian, A. & Stomph, M. (2009) *Diversity Matters: Guiding Principles on
      Diversity and Culture. W*orld Federation of Occupational Therapists
      (WFOT) Australia.

Swain, J., French, S., Barnes, C. & Thomas, C. (2004*) Disabling Barriers –
      Enabling Environments.*(2nd ed.) London: Sage.

Chapter 9: Patients' Perspective on Culture, Disability and Exercise: Perspectives from Nigeria

Adeonke Akinpelu, Nse Ayooluwa Odunaiya&Adesola Christiana Odole

Culture and Disability

Culture refers to a set of values and norms associated with a particular group, community, nation and society. It is a complex construct that cuts across the beliefs, values, customs, practices, social behaviour and artifacts that a society uses to cope with their world and with one another. These cultural attributes are transmitted from generation to generation through learning (Bates and Plog, 1991). All over the world, culture influences people's perception of disability.

Disability is common worldwide. The World Health Organization estimated that about 500 million people live with disability worldwide, 75% of them live in developing countries (Lang and Upah, 2008). Disability refers to limitations resulting from dysfunction in individual bodies and minds (Whyte and Ingstand, 2001). According to this bio-psychological definition, blindness, lameness, mental deficiency and chronic incapacitating illnesses are prototypical disabilities.

General Cultural Perspectives on Disability

According to Groce (1999), cultures view disability by its cause, by its effects on valued attributes and by the status of the disabled person as an adult. With regard to cause, people are treated well or poorly depending on cultural beliefs about how and why they became disabled. For instance, some cultures explain disability as resulting from witchcraft, reincarnation, divine displeasure, predestination and genetics. For example in Mexico and Botswana, the birth of a child with a disability is evidence of God's trust in a parent's ability to care for that child. With regard to effects of disability on valued attributes, if a society values physical strength, then people with physical disabilities are at a disadvantage. If a society values intellectual accomplishments, then the fact that a person uses a wheelchair is not a serious limitation to intellectual accomplishment. With regard to the disabled person's status as an adult, the willingness of a society to give resources to people with disabilities often depends on whether or not that individual will have an adult role in the community. Does that individual have a job, a family of his or her own? (Groce, 1999)

Disability is known to be a cause of poverty. According to Amusat, (2009), there is a strong relationship between disability and poverty, with cyclical tendency; poverty makes people more vulnerable to disability and disability reinforces and deepens poverty. People with disability are often excluded from mainstream of society and hence may not contribute to the development of the society at all or optimally. This vicious cycle of disability and poverty has been recognised and it led the United Nations to promulgate rules for equal opportunities for people with disability (United Nations, 1993). It also led to many international initiatives like those of the United Nations Educational, Scientific and Cultural Organization, the International Labour Organization and the World Health Organization (Amusat, 2009). The United Nations standard rules were supported by many countries. There is evidence that the implementation of the United Nations disability agenda has provided protection against discrimination for people with disability in the United Kingdom and improved the quality of life of people with disability in South Africa (Abatemi-Usman, 2013)..

Disability in Nigeria

Nigeria has roughly 12 million citizens who are disabled [United Nations, 2003]. This disabled population includes people with functional limitations due to physical, intellectual or sensory impairments, medical conditions or mental illness. A survey of 1093 persons with disabilities, conducted by the Leprosy Mission Nigeria in two (Kogi and Niger) of the thirty six states of Nigeria in 2005, reported that the most common disabilities involved vision (37%), mobility (32%) or hearing (15%). One third of the persons surveyed were less than 21 years old and had no occupations and 72% were Muslim. Over 50% had no education and the majority (61%were unemployed due to their disability (Smith, 2011). The author concluded that disability affects a person's ability to participate in education, work, family life and religion and contributes to poverty. Nigerian government promulgated a decree to enhance the social and societal position of people with disabilities in 1993 the law is definitely for the archives, and is not working (Amusat, 2009). Consequently, Nigerians with disabilities are still faced with the challenges of poverty, marginalization and exclusion despite the declaration of full participation in the disability agenda of the United Nations by the Nigerian government (Amusat, 2009). People with disability, especially in developing countries like Nigeria, irrespective of where they live, are more likely to be unemployed, illiterate, to have less formal education, and have less access to developed support networks and social capital than their able-body counterparts.

Nigerian Culture

The culture of Nigeria is shaped by its multiple ethnic groups. Nigeria has a population of about 150 million and more than 370 ethnic groups. The three major ethnic groups are Hausa-Fulani, the Igbo and the Yoruba. The Hausa-Fulani are predominantly in the north, the Igbo in the southeast and the Yoruba in the southwest. The Hausa-Fulani tend to be Muslim, the Igbo are predominantly Christian, while the Yoruba have a balance of members that adhere to both Islam and Christianity (Wikipedia, 2013). Indigenous religious practices remain important in all Nigeria ethnic groups and these beliefs are often blended with Christianity and Islam. Extended families are still the norm and are in fact the backbone of the social system. Grandparents, cousins, aunts, uncles, sisters, brothers and in-laws all work as a unit through life. Family relationships are guided by hierarchy and seniority. Social standing and recognition is achieved through extended families. Individuals turn to members of the extended family for financial aid and guidance, and the family is expected to provide for the welfare of every member. Although the role of the extended family is diminishing somewhat in urban areas, there remains a strong tradition of mutual caring and responsibility among the members (Wikipedia, 2013).

Perspective on Disability in the Nigerian Culture

People with disability are commonly perceived as being dependent, helpless and in need of charity. They are socially devalued and so faced stigmatizing attitudes that result in discrimination and segregation (Etuka, 2009). Consequently, people with disability in Nigeria are often faced with several challenges that militate against their social inclusion within contemporary society. These challenges include people's negative attitudes, institutional and environmental barriers Cultural beliefs about disability in many cultures therefore fuel the mutually negative symbiotic relationship between poverty and disability. The general perception of the Nigerian society to people with disability can be almost as varied as its ethnic, religious and cultural multiplicities (Alamu, 1992). The attitudes are generally negative and they differ from one part of the country to the other. The attitude ranges from viewing people with disability as pariahs to considering them as economic burden. Alamu (1992) summarized the attitudes of Nigerians to disability as follows:

   a.   "Send him out to beg": The practice of sending persons with disabilities to the street to beg for alms stems from the religious belief of some Nigerians that alms giving is a way of investing as well as waiving off temporal misfortunes. People with disabilities who live by begging become independent and often homeless. Through begging they are rejected, become homeless and miss out on the love of parents and later on spousal love
   b.   "I am ashamed of you": This attitude is implied through various reactions. People with disabilities are locked up at homes and sent to institutions, even when their disability constitutes no threat to anybody. Families do this probably for fear of being ridiculed by their neighbours and the public. When shut up this way, they are denied the normal

atmosphere for full development and opportunity to participate in normal activities such as educational, economic, political and social pursuits. In addition, this attitude has denied many people with mild disability of friendship and marital relationships. The attitude of "I am ashamed of you" often leads to frustration.

c. "It is not my business": This is an attitude of indifference, exemplified by sayings like "I thank God nobody is like this in my family". This is the rather callous posture assumed by many people and government of Nigeria. The impression is that the Nigerian society does not attach any importance to the lives of people with disability. The principle of responsible citizenship states that able-body citizens of any country should provide for the needs of their less-fortunate citizens, particularly, persons with disabilities. This attitude therefore deviates from that of a responsible society.

d. "He is worthless": Underneath this attitude is the supposition that what makes a person of any significance is the physical attributes. People with disabilities are regarded as worthless due to physical or mental impairments. The rate of ignorance of the Nigerian society regarding mental illness is high because it is often associated with supernatural causes such as break of a taboo or customs.

People with disability experience widespread discrimination and stigmatization as a result of these attitudes (Okafor, 2003). Stigmatization is a phenomenon where an individual reacts negatively to another person on the basis of a disability (Alamu, 1992). According to a Nigerian with disability (Chuks Etuka), getting admitted into a college was tough. Although he passed the entrance examination, he was told that he failed because of stigmatization and the assumption that I would not be able to cope with the other 'normal' students. He also reported that God touched the man in charge who later apologized and told him the truth that he passed very well (Etuka, 2009). People with disability are the least cared for in the Nigerian society. According to Chuks Etuka, the Nigeria society, due to cultural belief and ways of thinking has been very harsh to persons with disability and the government is not concerned and is unaccommodating towards persons with disability. Chuks Etuka believed that Nigerians perceive persons with disability as being sub-human, worthless and good-for-nothing. It is unfortunate, the Nigerian government has not done anything for persons with disability in anything; we are still being relegated to the background in everything (Etuka, 2009). Generally, families bear the brunt of caring for their members with disabilities throughout life. Those who cannot stay with their families are usually ostracised and their legal rights, including rights to live peacefully are threatened. People with physical disabilities in Nigeria have a heavy psychological burden due to social deprivations coupled with their struggle for economic survival (Okafor, 2003).

Perspective on Culture, Disability and Exercise in Nigeria—Patients' Narratives

In this sub topic, we present the narratives of adults and parents of children living with disabilities.Patients' [people with disability] perception on culture, disability and exercise are sparse in literature generally. In order to have empirical data to support what we know exist in our context, we explored patients' and proxies' perspective using focus group discussion and in-depth interview. A focus guide was developed. There was a moderator who led the discussion and an independent observer who recorded the discussion. Detailed information about the purpose and procedure of the focus group discussion/interview was provided. Participants were also informed that their voices would be recorded. They also assured of the confidentiality of all information they would provide. All patients and proxies gave consent. The focus groups comprised a group of four adults who have been living with physical disability from childhood and a group of three mothers and one grandmother of children with neuro-developmental delay. The physical disability of the adults was varying degrees of mobility limitation resulting from poliomyelitis infection. One of them was in a wheel chair, two used a pair of axillary crutches and the fourth person walked without any aid. Two of the children had cerebral palsy, one had spina bifida and one had Down's syndrome. Two persons with adult-onset physical disability resulting from stroke and excised spinal tumour were interviewed. Here is a summary of the themes of the study:

A. Perspective on Disability in the Nigerian Cultural Context
   1. Context of family support (sub-categories: parental attitude, siblings' attitude)
   2. Context of environment (sub-categories: accessibility, public transportation)
   3. Context of socialization (sub-categories: exclusion, stigmatization, segregation)
   4. Context of healthcare (sub-categories: attitude of healthcare professionals, healthcare professionals' communication skill, health education on long-term effects of disability on general health)
   5. Context of marriage (sub-category: late marriage and mal-adjustment in choice of marriage partner)
   6. Context of government policies (sub-category:non-implementation of government policy)

B. Perspective on Exercise in the Nigerian Culture
   1. Context of prescribed exercises (sub-category: effectiveness of exercise)
   2. Context of availability of exercise facilities

Perspectives on Disability in the Nigerian Cultural Context

Context of Family Support

Parental Attitude

This theme explored the impact of culture on family support for people with disability. All patients and proxies agreed that the family is the main source of support for people with disability in Nigeria. The family plays a very important role in individual perception of disability. A participant said:

> If your family sees you as a normal person and accepts you, then you can face the world with confidence and overcome many challenges that people with disability face.

According to the patients, parents' attitudes vary. Positive parental attitude gave three of the patients in the focus group the opportunity to get educated. A participant who did not receive this level of support from parent said:

> When I was young, I heard doctors advising my mother to register me in a primary school, but my mother was more interested in her trade. She dropped me in the village with my grandmother and I ended up not going to school. I am able to read the Yoruba bible because I had some form of adult education later.

Parents' attitudes were also influenced by the type of family setting. One patient from a polygamous setting reported that the father did not show any interest in his well being or education, but his mother gave him all the support he needed. He said:

> If not for my mother's support, I would not have been able to earn a living through honorable job as I now do

Another patient from a monogamous family setting reported that her father remained the source of her motivation in life because he is proud that I am a university graduate and a school teacher despite my physical disability. She said:

> My parent never hid me from members of our extended family or visitors. He would always invite me to our living room to be introduced to visitors.

The proxies agreed that mothers carry most of the burden of the care of children with disabilities, even when the fathers are supportive. A participant who is a grandmother among them reported that she has been staying with her daughter to relieve her of the burden for over one year. A participant who is a stroke survivor, an elderly woman in her eighties said that her children have been very supportive, although she still could not cope with the thought of having to be in a wheelchair on a permanent basis.

Siblings' Attitude

Patients from a monogamous family setting enjoyed the support of their siblings, whereas those from a polygamous setting reported that the attitude of their half siblings and step-mothers were negative. One of them said his half siblings looked down on him when he was young; he said "*I thank God because many of them now look up to me for counsel and financial assistance*".

Context of the Environment

Accessibility

This context explored patients' perception on the impact of the Nigerian environment on disability. All adult patients agreed that people living with physical disability encounter more environmental barriers in Nigeria than those living in many other countries of the world. Ambulating with walking aids or using a wheelchair on the road is difficult because of the absence of walkways. The risk of being knocked down by vehicles is high and the recently introduced commercial motorcycles increase the risk. In addition, ramps for wheelchair accessibility are not available in most public buildings, including banks, schools including institutions of higher learning, stadia and some hospitals. Many multi-storey buildings in Nigeria are built without lifts. In the few buildings with lifts, there is the risk of getting trapped in them because of the erratic nature of electricity supply in the country. The psychological impact of these environmental barriers on those with a disability is great. One patient said "*Attending institution of higher learning was tough for me. My choice of institution of higher learning was limited by environmental barrier. I read fine art and graphics in a polytechnic instead of a university where I was first offered admission because it was impossible for me to get to the fourth floor where the fine art studio was located in the university*".

Transportation

The public transport system in Nigeria does not make special provisions for people with disability. Big buses with facilities for easy accessibility by people in a wheelchair and those with walking aids are generally not available in Nigeria. In most towns in Nigeria, public transport is by cars and mini buses. One of the patients, who happened to be the chairman of an association for people with disability in Oyo State, observed that the routes plied by buses are not written on the buses and this makes travelling by public transport difficult for people with hearing disability. Transportation for people in a wheelchair is usually by special arrangement and is more expensive than normal. Some patients miss hospital appointments because of this difficulty. People with physical disabilities who use walking aids like crutches may have to struggle to get into the vehicle with able-body individuals during the "rush" hours to get to school or to work on time. One patient recounted his experience as follows: "*I attended a special primary school for people with disabilities in Lagos. The school bus would pick me at my doorstep. The struggle started when I gained admission to a secondary school and I had to get to school by public transport. I fell down a number of times, struggling to get inside the bus with able-body people during the "rush" hours. Eventually, I resolved to going late to school to avoid the "rush" hours".*

Context of Socialization

Exclusion

The needs of people with disability are not considered in many areas of life. Public buildings are constructed without consideration for easy accessibility by people with disability. The chairman of an association for people with disability reported that there was no one to communicate with a man with hearing disability once he accompanied him to a teaching hospital. A lady on crutches said a secretary once did not allow her to see the bank manager. She also reported that she intentionally arrived at a church before a wedding service started, but she was also told to wait outside and allow "real" people to come into a church for the wedding service. She reported that the experience was very frustrating.

Stigmatization

Nigerians with disability face a lot of stigmatization. Once you are in a wheelchair or you move around with a pair of crutches, you are more or less labeled a beggar. The elderly stroke survivor reported that she had to explain to people who offered her alms that she was not a beggar. One patient reported that out of ignorance, a co-tenant whom he once shared toilet facility with would scrub the shower with hot water and detergent to avoid being infected with my disability. Another one reported that she was once given a very inhumane reception when she was transferred to another school by the State teaching Service Commission. The reaction of the principal and the assistant principal of the secondary school to seeing a teacher walking with a pair of crutches was extremely negative, and they "politely" told her that her service was not needed. The lady said that she was bailed out of this embarrassing situation by a visiting teacher who testified that she was a very hard working teacher.

Segregation

Segregation is a major problem that people living with disability in Nigeria have to face. Two of the patients reported that landlords have refused to rent out accommodation to them because they were disabled. The reason given by one of the landlords is that people with disabilities would not be able to keep the accommodation clean, while the second landlord gave no reason. When you want to buy things in the open market, traders, thinking that you had come to beg for alms, might ask you to go away to allow others (able-bodied people) patronize them. The proxies reported that their children were not accepted in day care centres because of their disabilities. One mother said the reason given by a day care owner for refusing to accept her child was that other parents might stop bringing their children to the day care centre if they should see the child with disability in the centre.

Context of Healthcare

Attitude of Healthcare Professionals

In this context, we explored how the patients viewed the impact of healthcare on their disabilities in the Nigerian cultural context. According to the patients, no public hospital in Nigeria implements government policy on issuance of certificates to people with permanent disabilities or free health services for people with disability. There are no special considerations for people with disability in most public hospitals. A male patient in a wheelchair also said he once went to a hospital, spent the whole day moving up and down without being attended to. No assistance is available to families of people with disabilities to make structural adjustments at home in order to promote accessibility and independence of people with disability. Special rehabilitation centres are not available in Nigeria. Healthcare professionals do not appear to work together as a team; one would tell you one thing, another would tell you the opposite. While some healthcare professionals are caring and helpful, others are insensitive to the plight of people with disability. The story of a young female university graduate with adult onset disability who was in a wheelchair summarizes the impact of healthcare professionals' attitude on disability. She said *"Nigerian healthcare culture has messed up the minds of many people with disability. Imagine a neurosurgeon who has been managing people like me telling me, just before discharge from hospital to go home, eat and enjoy your life; there is nothing to bother about, no one would employ you. This threw me into more confusion and depression. I wondered what the future had for me. My parents were even more confused and requested that I should be allowed to stay longer in the hospital because they had no clue as to how to handle me at home after discharge. However, one of the physiotherapists who managed me introduced me to another young lady with similar problem. The lady counseled me and motivated me to face the challenges of living with disability. This helped me overcome depression, gained good level of independence. I eventually got employed by a teaching hospital as an administrator. My parents tell me every time that they have been encouraged by my attitude and the way I cope with my disability"*.

Healthcare Professionals' Communication Skill

Patients reported that they were not given detailed information about their conditions, but they were left on their own to discover the permanent nature of their disabilities and the challenges ahead of them. Proxies reported that they were not given detailed information about the cause of their children's disabilities; two of them attributed the cause to some evil power. One mother said she was given false hope by some health workers who assured her that her child would soon gain head control, but the child has not after almost three years. A lady said *"After surgery and removal of the catheter, I woke up one day to find myself in a pool of urine and faeces. I asked the nurses in the ward to explain what happened to me, but they advised me to talk to the surgeons. At the end, I discovered on my own that my being unable to control urine and faeces was a complication of the surgery I had. It was a most frustrating experience that none of healthcare professionals in charge of my care was ready to explain the problem to me"*.

Health Education on Long-term Effects of Disability on General Health

Patients with mobility problem secondary to poliomyelitis infection in childhood complained that they were not educated about the long term effects of their disability. One of them said he knew about post-polio syndrome only recently. Another one reported that no one told him that the risk of obesity is high in people in a wheelchair.

Context of Marriage

Late Marriage and Mal-adjustment in the Choice of a Marriage Partner

In this context, we explored the effect of disability on the patients' chances of getting married. Disability reduces the chances of getting married as well as choices of life partners. One lady in her forties reported she was not married yet because of lack of suitor. A male patient reported that he could not marry an able-body lady he was in love with because her parents and family members did not endorse their relationship. He resorted to marrying a lady with physical disability. Another young lady said she married the only man who was interested in her, a Muslim even though she is a Christian. She said, *"If I had a choice, I would marry a Christian but none was interested in me because of my disability. I thank God because I am a mother of two children"*.

Context of GovernmentPolicies

Non-implementation of GovernmentPolicy

In this context, we investigated the patients' views on the implementation of the policy contained in the Nigerians with Disabilities Decree of 1993 and how it has influenced their well being. All the patients agreed that most aspects the government policy remained unimplemented twenty years after the decree was promulgated. According to the patients, public hospitals do not provide free healthcare services to people with disabilities in Nigeria. The few vocational training centres established by government lack adequate facilities and personnel. Some of these centres are sometimes used as camps for the destitute. People with disabilities are not provided with housing subsidies. Vehicles used for public transportation are not fitted with facilities to ease accessibility. The effect of the non-implementation of the policy is that people with disabilities in Nigeria are still confronted with many challenges which their counterparts in developed countries do not face.

Perspective on Exercisein the Nigerian Culture

Context of Prescribed Exercises

In this theme, we explored the views of the patients and proxies on the effectiveness of the therapeutic exercises they or their children/grandchild are taken through in the hospital.

Effectiveness of Exercises

All the patients and proxies agreed that therapeutic exercises have been useful in improving their functional performance. One proxy said, *"My child's head control has improved since he started physiotherapy"*. However, one mother reported that she has not observed any improvement in her child's functional performance since he started physiotherapy about six months ago. All the four patients with childhood onset disability reported that they stopped attending physiotherapy clinics many years ago, partly out of ignorance and partly due to their struggle for survival. They reported that they were privileged to participate in an arm ergometric exercise training organized by a research student recently and they benefitted a lot from it. According to them, the exercise programme was an eye opener and they wished that such exercise training programme could be made available to people with mobility disability, even if they have to pay a token for it. The school teacher among them said *"Unlike before the arm ergometric exercise training, I now stand (supported with my crutches) throughout morning assembly in my school. I have also lost over five-kilogramme weight, I feel lighter and my body is in the 'up and go' state"*. Some of the patients and the proxies however reported that they were not given specific exercises as home assignment. Those who were given exercise home assignment were not given detailed instructions about repetition and frequency of the exercises. In response to a question asked on how their exercises were progressed, a patient reported that the exercises prescribed for her are not varied or progressed. She said *"I have been going through the same set of exercises for many weeks; I find them boring. I continue attending physiotherapy clinic because I do not want my legs to become thin"*

Context of Availability of Exercise Facilities

The patients reported that facilities for exercise and sports are not readily available, even for able-bodied people in their neighborhood. According to them, this might be partly responsible for the general poor exercise habit of the average Nigerian. One of them recalled that in special school for physically challenged which he attended as a child, students were going for swimming regularly and that there were floating accessories to assist them with the exercise.

Conclusion and Implications from the Patients' Narratives

From the narratives, major issues with regard to Nigerian culture, disability and exercise have been identified. There are challenges to tackle both by the healthcare professionals and the government. There is a strong need for acculturation within the family and the society at large. The issues identified are:

1. Ignorance of the Nigerian populace on causes and impact of disability on individuals living with disabilities.
2. Healthcare providers' negative attitude and poor communication skills in managing these individuals living with disabilities.

3. Non-implementation of government policy on the rights and mainstreaming of individuals living with disabilities.
4. Therapeutic exercises though appreciated by individuals living with disabilities for their beneficial effects, are not adequately monitored and progressed.

We believe that all these challenges could be addressed primarily by implementation of government policy, education of healthcare professionals on disability and effective communication, inclusion of disability as a subject in school curriculum at all levels and acculturation of family units and larger society.

References

Abatemi-Usman, N. 2013. A case for Nigerians living with with disabilities. The National Mirror, February 11 & 12, 2013.

Alamu, J. F. 1992. The plight of the disabled in Nigeria and what can be done. Lagos; Wellsprings Publications pages 8-18.

Amusat, N (2009) Disability Care in Nigeria: The need for professional advocacy. African Journal of Physiotherapy and Rehabilitation 1: 30-36.

Bates, D. G., Plog, F. 1991 as cited by Eldey D. G., Robey K. L. 2005. Considering the culture of disability in cultural competence education. Academic Medicine 80 (7): 706-712.

Etuka, C. 2009. Chuks Etuka and his will to survive. Viewed May 1, 2013. http://nigeriavillagesquare.com/articles/ahaoma-kanu/chuks-etuka-and-his-will-to-survive-12.html.

Groce, N. E. 1999. Disability in cross-cultural perspective: Rethinking disability. *The Lancet 354:* 756-757.

Lang, R., Upah L. 2008. Scoping Study: Disability issues in Nigeria. Viewed April 29, 2013. http://www.ucl.ac.uk/lcccr/downloads/dfidnigeriareport

Okafor, L. 2003. Enhancing business-community relationships: Sir David Osunde Foundation case study. Viewed May 12, 2013, http://www.worldvolunteerweb.org/fileadmin/docs/old/pdf/2003/031201_EBCR_NGA_davidosunde.pdf

Smith, N (2011) The face of disability in Nigeria: A disability survey in Kogi and Niger States. Disability, CBR and Inclusive Development, 22 (1) (Dio10.5463/DCID.v11i22.11)

The Guardian. 2009. Nigerian amputated in Sierra Leone devotes life helping the disabled. April 12, 2009.

United Nations (1993) UN standard rules on equalization of opportunities for people with disabilities. Viewed May 1, 2013 http://www.wcpt.org/node/29219.

United Nations population and vital statistics report. 2003. Viewed April, 29, 2013. http://unstats.un.org/unsd/disability/disform.asp

Whyte, SR, Ingstand, B 2001. Disability and Culture: An Overview. Viewed May 5, 2013 http://books.google.com.ng/books?hl=en&lr=&id=750iSwBZBmkC&oi=fnd&pg=PA3&dq=disability+and+culture+an+overview&ots=7VBET EDVRT&sig=bG0XgD1Fe3fllodjZFv-20TL-

94&redir_esc=y#v=onepage&q=disability%20and%20culture%20an%2
0overview&f=false
Wikipedia. Nigerian culture. Viewed May 12, 2013.
http://en.wikipedia.org/wiki/Culture_of_Nigeria

Chapter 10: Cultural Competence and Disability: A Lifelong Journey to Cultural Proficiency, Part II

Ronnie Leavitt

Introduction

This chapter hopes to convince rehabilitation professionals to be more oriented to socio-cultural domains; areas that are typically found within the social science and public policy arenas. This includes a greater appreciation of material conditions, social relationships, and aspects of the non-material culture (i.e. values and beliefs): such as ethnicity, disability status, economic status, political environment, religion, gender, sexuality, and other similar variables that clinicians often ignore. With greater insight into the variation of social, cultural, and economic conditions that others experience, attempts to improve the life situation of our clients are likely to be more successful. At the same time, if rehabilitation professionals truly consider social and cultural domains, social scientists are likely to pay more attention to people with disability.

In this chapter I will also consider broad categories as a starting point from which to delve deeper into the life of the individual patient. One should not generalize about an entire disability or ethnic group anymore than a health professional would generalize about a patient with a stroke or Parkinson's disease. A health professional would ask a multitude of questions and keenly observe the patient for clues to the person's full situation. If a client came to you with a diagnosis with which you were unfamiliar, you would access information about the problem to learn more. Similarly, it is appropriate to access information about the client's cultural ways of life if those are not familiar to you. This chapter will look at these issues.

Cultural Competence and 'Evidence-Based Practice', 'Patient-Centred Care', and Ethical Decision Making

The health professions are promoting "evidence-based practice", (EBP), in clinical decision-making. This concept presumes ..." 'open and thoughtful clinical decision-making' about the ...management of a patient/client that integrates the 'best available evidence with clinical judgment' and the patient/client's preferences and values, and that further considers the larger social context in which ... services are provided, to optimize patient/client outcomes and quality of life." (Jewell 2008 p.8). Thus, within the definition itself, the socio-cultural context is recognized as being important. According to Jewell (2008), once the validity of a test/ measure or treatment is established one must still consider whether the evidence is appropriate for use with a given patient. It is at this time that the clinician will consider personal expertise and judgment in addition to the patient preferences and values. For example, the cultural and social norms for the patient/family may affect the feasibility of a particular intervention. Therefore, the challenge is to collect evidence from three sources. The final decision making process is based on these factors: research-based clinical evidence, clinician judgment, and patient need.

Cultural competence also considers "patient-centered care", another emerging bedrock principle when delivering health care. This is "characterized by informed, shared decision-making, development of patient knowledge, skills needed for self-management of illness, and preventive behaviors." Patients' and families need an opportunity to have input on preferences and values. According to Knebel in (2008), patient-centered care rejects the traditionally practiced bio-medical model whereby health care professionals alone, based solely on "scientific" evidence, make decisions *for* the patient without consideration of a shared decision-making partnership *with* the patient and taking into account their unique perspective and their way of life.

With regard to the broader domain of health care, health professionals are duty bound to accept the major health care ethical principles of autonomy, beneficence, and justice (Morrison 2009). Based on a review of the cultural value systems associated with different populations, (See Leavitt, 2010, chapter 1 for more detail), it is possible to imagine how ideas concerning these ethical principles might not be the same for different people. For example, autonomy may be held in high esteem by people from individualistic cultures and potentially not much at all in a collectivist culture. Also, paternalism, gender inequality or the valuing of elders, may affect who makes a decision for someone in the family. The idea of telling the truth to a patient, something that Euro-American health professionals are taught, may be secondary to allowing someone to "save face". What if, according to the principle of self-determination, a patient refuses a treatment that they really know very little about? What is considered evil or good are certainly not universal concepts. In a hierarchical society, concern for justice may be deemed not important as compared to a society that thinks of itself as egalitarian. One of the real challenges, therefore, facing someone who is working toward becoming culturally competent is the ability to evaluate a situation without focusing solely on their own ethical perspective and decision-making process. Practitioners must recognize the challenge to ethnocentrism and the potential for inherent conflicts.

More Definitions

As healthcare professionals from various disciplines recognize the importance of cultural competence in the delivery of culturally appropriate health care, the theoretical models and conceptual frameworks describing this domain have evolved. There are a range of associated definitions, models, assessment and measurement tools. Some of these are described below to demonstrate the variability in the approach to thinking about cultural competence and the variability of methods to attempt to measure cultural competence for an individual or organization. It can be useful to determine which of the selected ideas and methods are really most useful and practical for you.

Definitions of Key Concepts Associated with Cultural Competence

As noted above, Cross et al (1989) have developed the most widely utilized definition and framework for understanding the meaning of cultural competence. Additional commonly used terms are described here, although the evolutionary nature of the concept requires that definitions and meanings will continue to develop. Some are used interchangeable, such as cross-cultural, trans-cultural, and intercultural.

Cultural diversity assumes that people are different. This assumption has been used to simplify the presence of human variation within the health care system. There has been a history of providing 'cultural diversity' education, generally focusing on cultural awareness and cultural knowledge by giving information about specific groups of people. Recognizing diversity and diverse ways to live life or receive health care, although a first step, does nothing to meet the varying needs of diverse peoples; knowledge alone does not necessarily translate into action.

The term *multicultural* assumes that a culture is heterogeneous with regard to age, color, ethnicity, gender, national origin, political ideology, race, religion, and sexual orientation—and includes the presence and participation of people with disabilities and those from different socioeconomic backgrounds. Typically, practitioners accept today's reality of "living in a multicultural world" or supporting the concept of a "multicultural environment". But, the concept must use the sensitivity, knowledge and skill development and adaptation components of cultural competence to effect meaningful changes in a world composed of individuals with diverse ideas, perspectives, and backgrounds.

Medical pluralism suggests that in every society, although there may be a predominant system for delivering health care, alternative systems exist simultaneously. It may also recognize that a single entity (person or family) may pick and choose elements of a range of systems. For example, in 1993, Eisenberg et al published the first comprehensive American survey describing the use of complientary and alternative medical therapies (CAM); i.e. defined as those healthcare and medical practices that are not currently an integral part of conventional medicine. At that time, approximately one third of adults in the USA had used at least one CAM during the last year. A follow-up survey in 1997 concluded that 42% of the population used CAM (Eisenberg et al 1998). This number has almost certainly gone up.

Culturally congruent care, a term initiated by Leininger (1991) is defined as "those cognitively based assistive, supportive, facilitative, or enabling acts or decisions that are tailor made to fit with individual, group, or institutional cultural values, beliefs, and lifeways in order to provide or support meaningful, beneficial, and satisfying health care or well-being services." Culturally congruent care can occur only if one knows, and uses in a meaningful and appropriate way, the values, expressions, patterns, and practices of culturally diverse groups and individuals.

New terms continue to enter the cultural competence lexicon. *Cultural humility* (Tervalon & Murray-Garcia 1998) has been defined as a commitment to make the life-long journey toward cultural proficiency through self-critique and action toward changing the power imbalances in the client-health care professional relationship. Nunez (2000) has suggested the term *cross-cultural efficacy* to represent the ability of a caregiver to be effective in interactions that involve individuals of different cultures by ensuring that neither the caregivers' nor patients' culture is the preferred or the more accurate view.

Fisher et al (2007) have coined the term *cultural leverage* when designing and implementing culturally congruent interventions. That is "a focused strategy for improving the health of racial and ethnic communities by using their cultural practices, products, philosophies, or environments as vehicles that facilitate behavior change of patients and practitioners" (Fischer 2007, p. 245S).

Never the less, the term *cultural competence* has taken hold most often as advocates for a better approach to care realize its more encompassing nature. The goal of moving towards cultural proficiency, the last stage of cultural competence on Cross et al's (1989) continuum should be our objective.

Eliciting Cultural Information Using Patient-centred Models

In contrast to the theoretical models discussed in chapter 6 defining cultural competence and/ or focusing on the process by which health professionals can become culturally competent, other models are more patient-centred and require gaining knowledge about what people think, feel, want, and need. They emphasize the insider's point of view known as an *emic* approach. This is in contrast to the *etic* or outsider's point of view.

The Purnell Model for Cultural Competence (Purnell and Palunka 2003) is an organizing framework to assess cultural values, beliefs, behaviors, and healthcare practices of individuals. It is a holistic model applicable for a range of providers but not all of the components are directly applicable to all types of health care practice. Nevertheless, recognition of the global society (eg. world politics/ conflicts; natural disasters; business practices; and more), community (a group of people having a common interest or identity through physical or social connections), family (eg. physically or socially connected individuals), and person (a biological, psychological, sociological, cultural being) as well as the broad range of interconnected domains enumerated assist one to think broadly in working toward cultural proficiency.

Leininger (1993) uses a "sunrise" graphic to describe her Theory of Culture Care Diversity and Universality. She identifies the influence of seven cultural and social structure dimensions on a person's well-being. These are:

1. Cultural values and lifeways
2. Religious, philosophical, and spiritual beliefs
3. Economic factors
4. Educational factors
5. Technological factors
6. Kinship and social ties
7. Political and legal factors.

Leininger (1993) suggests that information gleaned about the above domains should be used by the provider to guide their selection of approach(es). This guidance can occur through 1) cultural care preservation; 2) cultural care accommodation; and 3) cultural care restructuring if a cultural practice is deemed detrimental to health (Leininger 1993).

Giger and Davidhizar (2002) posit that cultural competence is a dynamic, fluid, continuous process whereby an individual, system, or agency finds useful and meaningful strategies to deliver care based on knowledge of the cultural heritage, attitudes, and behaviors of those to whom care is delivered. Their Transcultural Assessment Model asks questions focusing on how six factors can influence health beliefs and practices. The six cultural phenomena to be considered are: (1) communication (verbal and non-verbal style), (2) space (personal boundaries), (3) social organization (family structure and religious values), (4) time (time reckoning and consideration of past, present and future), (5) environmental control (health practices), and (6) biological variation (physical attributes, nutritional preferences, and diseases specific to their cultural group).

Related to the patient-centered models that explore specific domains of culture, others focus on a more general approach about what questions the provider should ask and 'how to" ask them. The following are some of the more commonly used guides to elicit socio-cultural information from a patient.

Arguably the most well-known concept is that of the Explanatory Model (EM), defined by Kleinman (1980). Open-ended questions are used to allow patients to discuss their health, based on their perceptions of a particular illness or condition (i.e. and *emic* approach). The clinician should ask the patient questions such as:

- What do you call your problem?
- What do you think caused your problem?
- What are the greatest problems your illness has caused for you?
- What do you fear most about the consequences of this illness?
- What kind of treatment do you think you should receive?
- What are the most important results you hope to get from your treatment?

Kleinman (1980) reminds health care professionals that although we need to focus on the patient's EM, it is essential to understand that clinicians also have an EM and operate within their own distinct culture. The patient and his or her family cannot be expected to always and completely comply with the practitioner's EM, and the health care professional cannot be expected to "buy into" the patient's.

Additionally, there are a range of useful mnemonics for assessing a client's culture or when trying to skillfully gather patient information. These mnemonics generally intend to foster respect for client centrality, avoid stereotyping, and allow for adoption of mutually acceptable ways to encourage success. None are the best for all situations.

Berlin and Fowkes (1982) have suggested using the mnemonic LEARN when assessing your patient's culture:

> Listen to the client's perception of the problem.
> Explain your perception of the problem from a health professional point of view.
> Acknowledge the similarities and differences between the two perceptions.
> Recommend a plan of care that takes into account the patient's perceptions and builds upon similarity of ideas as much as possible.
> Negotiate a treatment plan that can work for both parties and realistically be carried out.

Alternatively, Stuart and Lieberman (1993) suggest the mnemonic BATHE for eliciting the patient's psychological context with regard to their visit to the health professional. The following are the suggested questions:

> Background – What is going on in your life?
> Affect – How do you feel about what is going on?
> Trouble – What about the situation troubles you the most?
> Handling – What are you doing about the problem?
> Empathy – The provider should offer psychological support.

Measuring Cultural Competence: A Challenge

There are many challenges to measuring the elements of cultural competence that make it difficult to use concrete measurement tools to capture the relationship of culture to an individual, organization, health care delivery system, and society. The many factors influencing health related outcomes makes it difficult to isolate the contribution of cultural competence and is outside the scope of this chapter. (See Leavitt 2010, chapter 3 for more information)

Self-assessment of Cultural Competence by Health Professionals

Many self-assessment tools help individuals and agencies examine their cultural and linguistic competence. Self-assessments have inherent limitations, yet they are also beneficial for gathering information to begin a life-long process of creating more awareness, knowledge, and skills. A large number of instruments have been used in the nursing, mental health and social work professions to measure one or more constructs of cultural *competence, although many do not have data supporting their reliability and* validity (Roziner 1996). None are specific to cultural competence for particular disability groups. Selected tools are listed here.

A literature review indicates that most titles associated with cultural competence assessment are actually recommended check-off lists of personal, departmental or organizational characteristics and activities that can be considered in determining the degree of cultural competence.(See Leavitt 2010, chapter 12 for examples.)Personal style and work place requirements will influence decisions regarding which of these to use.

The Cultural Competence Health Practitioner Assessment (CCHPA) is a self-assessment tool to promote better delivery of health care services to culturally and linguistically diverse people and underserved communities. The CCHPA measures data in six subscales: values and belief systems; cultural aspects of epidemiology; clinical decision-making; life cycle events; cross-cultural communication; and empowerment/ health management (CCHPA accessed Nov. 19, 2008). It takes approximately 20 minutes to complete.

Shim et al (2003) and Doorenbos et al (2005) have developed the cultural competence assessment instrument (CCA). The CCA has an internal consistency reliability of 0.89 overall, with 0.91 and 0.75 for the two subscales. Construct validity was supported and mean scores were significantly higher for providers who reported previous diversity training compared to those who had not.

Arguably, the most used instrument to measure cultural competence is that developed by Campinha-Bacote (2003). The Inventory for Assessing The Process of Cultural Competence Among Healthcare Professionals – Revised (IAPCC-R) measures the level of cultural competence among health professionals. It is a self-administered tool consisting of 25 items that measure five cultural constructs in a model of desire awareness, knowledge, skill, and encounters. Scores are based on a 4-point Likert scale, with higher scores indicating greater competence. Content validity has been established by national experts and reliability has been calculated by coefficient Cronbach alpha scores of .85 and .90 for two groups of nurses.

The newest version of the IAPCC is the IAPCC-SV to measure the level of cultural competence among students in health professions (Campinha-Bacote 2007). It consists of 20 items measuring the five cultural constructs on a 4-point Likert scale. Content validity was established by national expert review and reliability testing demonstrated a Cronbach's alpha of .783 (Fitzgerald et al 2007).

Among other self-assessment scales measuring different aspects of cultural competence that have demonstrated moderate or better internal consistency and reliability (Cronbach's alpha coefficients of >0.70) include the Cross Cultural Adaptability Inventory (CCAI) (Kelley and Meyers 1992), the Multicultural Awareness-Knowledge- and Skills Assessment (MAKSS) developed byD'Andrea, Daniels, and Heck (1991) the Multicultural Counseling Inventory (MCI) (Sodowsky et al 1994),the Cultural Self-Efficacy Scale (CSES) (Smith 2001), and the Self-Assessment Questionnaire (CCSAQ) (Mason 1995).

The critical question of the degree to which an individual moves toward cultural competence and cultural proficiency remains murky. Pope-Davis et al (1993) looking at occupational therapists found higher scores for those with higher levels of education and work experience with diverse populations or those who have taken courses related to multiculturalism. Similarly, Pope-Davis and Ottavi (1994) found that nursing students who had worked with a diverse population scored higher on a multicultural sensitivity and knowledge scale compared to students' without such experience.

In "Assessing the Impact of Cultural Competency Training using Participatory Quality Improvement Methods", Like et al (2004) note that physicians' self-perceived cultural competence knowledge, skill, and comfort levels improved significantly over time. However, the lack of experimental design or control did not allow the authors to conclude that it was the training intervention per se that caused the changes. The authors did suggest that quality improvement teams may improve providing culturally responsive care in clinical settings.

In the USA, the Association of American Medical Colleges (AAMC) has developed a Tool for Assessing Cultural Competence Training (TACCT) as part of a comprehensive curricular needs assessment for medical schools. The TACCT consists of 67 items measuring knowledge, skill or attitude. Lie et al 2006).

Still, it is generally believed that increased cultural knowledge without concurrent changes in attitudes and behavior is of limited value It may even prove harmful if stereotypes are merely reinforced (Tervalon and Murray-Garcia 1998). It seems that a lifelong commitment to self-evaluation and critique in order to develop mutually beneficial health care partnerships and achieve cultural proficiency is required (Tervalon and Murray-Garcia 1998, Cross et al 1989).

In sum, the conclusion of Brach and Fraser (2000) seems most accurate. Rigorous research on cultural competency techniques and outcomes is lacking. That is, "… while there is substantial research evidence to suggest that cultural competency should in fact work, heath systems have little evidence about which cultural competency techniques are effective and less evidence on when and how to implement them properly". (p.181)

Cultural Competence and Disability: Some Examples

As with all cultural groups the complex culture of disability needs to be an important consideration. Disability exists in all societies, yet how much does the casual observer (or even rehabilitation professionals) understand about the meaning of disability? How does one ever understand the lived experiences of persons with disabilities (PWD)? Broader appreciation of the reality of living with a disability (i.e. a consideration of all the previously mentioned variables such as socioeconomic status, health beliefs and health related behaviors, political environment, language, etc.) is rare among any health care professional, including those who may consider themselves disability advocates. Cultural competence, therefore, is an essential component of our professional lives.

This book addresses many topics associated with the culture of disability. Therefore, only a few practical examples, directly related to the notion of cultural competence will be provided here (See Leavitt 2010, chapter 5 for more information).

Once again, health professionals should not make sweeping generalizations, but must look for *intracultural* diversity. The assumption should be that a client with a disability will, in addition, have many other primary and secondary cultural characteristics that are also relevant in defining who that person is. The sub-culture of disability may be, more or less, salient for an individual or group. People with a disability may identify with only those with a similar diagnosis or those with a similar functional impairment. For example, people with hearing impairments often primarily identify with "the deaf community" (culture) and deafness may be one's major identifying factor. Deafness is not viewed as a limitation, rather a biological characteristic that has given rise to a specific culture and the slogans of "deaf pride" and "disability pride" (Groce 1999; Ravaud and Stiker 2001).

In the field of rehabilitation, it is especially critical to understand one's world view and/or value system. For example, the core values of a Euro-American physical therapist are likely to include individualism, and a value for youthfulness. In contrast, core values held by people of Asian or Hispanic descent (and others) emphasize collectivism (placing family first), and great respect for elders. Children must remain ever loyal for the sacrifices their parents made and are expected to provide financial, emotional and practical support for their parents. The clinician must consider how these core values will affect one's disability status and/or the rehabilitation process. Patient independence, valued so highly by Euro-American health care professionals may not be the goal. Religion is also relevant and closely allied to one's world view. Most clinicians in the USA and Europe will be Christian, but many Asian clients will be Buddhist. Buddhism views pain and suffering as a part of life, not to be complained about and the patient may not report discomfort to the healer (Leavitt 2003; Ling 2003).

Language barriers may be compounded by a person's disability status. In addition to the potential expected verbal and non-verbal style differences between and within cultural groups Having a disability may also affect spatial distancing and touch among other cultural characteristicsThese cultural characteristics should be considered further in the presence of a disability. For example, a PWD should be greeted with the same respect as someone without a disability. If an individual has difficulty greeting someone with a typical handshake, it is appropriate to reach out to the patient's right hand or shake the left hand. Or, if someone is in a wheelchair, it is important to sit, making "eye to eye" contact easier.

There is a significant variation in the cultural attitudes and beliefs about disability at the individual and family level (Antonek and Livneh 1988, Aiken 2002, Tervo et al 2002). Westbrook et al (1993), investigates the differences in the attitudes of six cultural groups in Australia with regard to 20 diagnoses. Overall, PWD was most accepted by the German community followed by the Anglo, Italian, Chinese, Greek and Arabic groups. Interestingly, the results did not show significant differences with regard to the concept of stigma hierarchy: in all communities, people with asthma, diabetes, heart disease and arthritis were the most accepted, and people with AIDS, mental retardation, psychiatric illness, and cerebral palsy, were the least. A greater discussion of this topic is found in Leavitt 2010, chapter 5 and other chapters in this book.

At the societal level, although there is intercultural and intracultural variations, three major categories of social beliefs seem to exist cross-culturally and tend to predict how well a PWD will fare in a particular community. These are: valued and disvalued attributes of the society, causality of the disability, and anticipated role for the person with the disability (Groce 1999). Cultural responses to the presence of disability at the individual, family, and societal level are equally varied. Behaviors or actions that occur typically result from the above beliefs and are in part secondary to material realities (See Leavitt 2010, chapter 5 and other chapters in this text).

Conclusion

The future is likely to see an increasing number of people with disabilities (PWD) from a range of cultural groups. It is presumed that there will be PWD in every society and that there will be specific medical care and socio-cultural systems and explanatory models that account for the beliefs about the disability and the cultural patterns of behaviours having to do with disability diagnosis and treatment. The social construction of disability is related in part to the influence of belonging to multiple cultural sub-groups, societal attitudes toward disability, the material realities of the environment, and the adaptation mechanisms that are available for any individual and their family. In removing barriers, disability rights activists will undoubtedly play a major role. Advancement of cultural competence by health professionals is necessary as well. Paradigms focusing on a client or family-centred model, including community based rehabilitation (CBR) and independent living, require paying attention to the client and their family's socio-cultural environment.

References

Aiken, LR 2002 *Attitudes and related psychosocial constructs: theories, assessment, and research.* Thousand Oaks, CA. Sage Pub.

Antonek, R. and Livneh, H. 1988 *The Measurement of Attitudes Toward People with Disabilities: Methods, Psychometrics and Scales.* Springfield IL: Charles C Thomas.

Bennett, M. J., (1993). Towards ethnorelativism: A developmental model of intercultural sensitivity. In R. M. Paige (ed.) Education for the intercultural experience. Yarmouth, ME: Intercultural Press

Berlin, EA and Foukes, WC. (1983) Teaching framework for cross cultural care : implications in family practice, *West J Med,* 139 (6) 934-938.

Borkan, J. & Neher, J (1991)*A developmental model of ethnicity in family practice training. Family Medicine,* 23 (3), 212-217.

Brach. C., Fraser I. 2000. Can cultural competency reduce racial and ethnic health disparities? A review and conceptual model. USDHHS, PHS, Agency for Healthcare

Research and Quality. AHRQ Publication No. 01-R007, Nov. 2000 in Medical Care Research and Review, Vol 57, Supplement 1, 181-217.

Campinha-Bacote, J. The Process of Cultural Competence in the Delivery of Healthcare Services. 2003. Transcultural C. A. R. E. Assoc.

Campinha-Bacote, J. The Process of Cultural Competence in the Delivery of Healthcare Services: The Journey Continues, 5th edition (2007)

Cross TL, Bazron BJ, Dennis KW, Isaacs MR. *Towards a Culturally Competent System of Care: A Monograph on Effective Services for Minority*

Children Who Are Severely Emotionally Disturbed. Vol 1. Washington, DC: Georgetown University, National Technical Assistance Center for Children's Mental Health; 1989.

Cultural Competence Health Practitioner Assessment (CCHPA), https://www4.georgetown.edu/uis/keybridge/keyform/form.cfm?formalI D=277

Accessed Nov. 19, 2008

D'Andrea, M., Daniels, J., Heck, R. (1991). Evaluating the impact of multicultural counseling training. J of Counseling and Development, 70, 143-150.

Doorenboos, A., Schim S., Benkert R., Borse, N. 2005. Psychometric evaluation of the cultural competence assessment instrument among health care providers. Nursing Research , Sept-Oct. 2005.

Eisenberg, D., Kessler R., Foster C. (1993). Unconventional medicine in the United States. NEJM 328, 246-252.

Eisenberg, D., Davis R., Ettner S., Appel S., Wilkey S., Van Rompey M., (1998). Trends in alternative medicineuse in the United States, 1990-1997. Journal of American medical Association, 280(18), 1569-1575.

Fisher, TL, Burnet DL, Huang ES, Chin MH, Cagney KA. Cultural leverage: interventions using culture to narrow racial disparities in health care. Med Care Res Rev2007 Oct; 64(5) Suppl: 243S-82S.

Fitzgerald, E. Cronin, S. and Campinha-Bacote, J. Psychometric Testing of the Inventory for Assessing the Process of Cultural Competence Among Healthcare Professionals-Student Version (IAPCC-SV) 2007.

Giger, J. N. and Davidhizar, R. ?2002. The Giger and Davidhizar transcultural assessment model. J of Transcultural Nursing, 13, 185-188.

Groce, N 1999 *Health beliefs and behavior towards individuals with disability cross-culturally* In: ed. Leavitt R Cross-Cultural Rehabilitation: An International Perspective. London: W. B. Saunders. Pp.37-48.

Jewell, Dianne 2008 Guide to Evidence-Based Physical Therapy Practice. Jones and Bartlett Pub. Sudbury, MA.

Kelley, C., Meyers J. 1992 Cross-cultural adaptability inventory manual. Minneapolis, Minn: NCS Pearon Inc.

Kleinman, A. *Patients and Healers in the Context of Culture: An Exploration of the Borderland Between Anthropology, Medicine, and Psychiatry.* Berkley, Calif: University of California Press; 1980.

Knebel, E. Educating Health Professionals to be Patient-Centered. Institute of Medicine Web site, http://www.iom.edu/Object. File/Master/10/460/Patient. Accessed Nov. 15, 2008.

Leavitt, RL, ed. 1999 *Cross-Cultural Rehabilitation: An International Perspective.* London, England: WB Saunders Co.

Leavitt, R 2003 *Developing cultural competence in a multicultural world.*PT Magazine Jan. pp.56-69.

Leavitt, R 2010 *Cultural competence: a lifelong journey to cultural proficiency.* Thorofare New Jersey: Slack Inc.

Leininger M (1993 winter) Towards conceptualization of transcultural health care systems: concepts and a model. J of Transcultural Nursing , 4 (2) 32-40.

Lie, D., Boker J., Cleveland, E. 2006. Using the tool for assessing cultural competence training (TACCT) to measure faculty and medical student perceptions of cultural competence instruction in the first three years of the curriculum. Academic Medicine, Vol. 81, No. 6, June 2006, pp. 557-564.

Like, R., Fulcomer, M., Kairys, J., Wathington, K., Crosson, J. 2004. Assessing the impact of cultural competency training using participatory quality improvement methods. Center for Health Families and Cultural Diversity Department of Family Medicine, University of Medicine and Dentistry of New Jersey (UMDNJ) – Robert Wood Johnson Medical School.

Ling, W 2003 *Cultural diversity of older Americans: an overview of East Asian cultures for physical therapists.* APTA, Section on Geriatrics, Home Study Course.

Loveland, C. The concept of culture. In: Leavitt RL, ed. *Cross-Cultural Rehabilitation: An International Perspective.* London, England: WB Saunders Co; 1999:15–24.

Lynch, EW, Hanson, MJ, eds. *Developing Cross-Cultural Competence: A Guide for Working With Young Children and Their Families.* 2nd ed. Baltimore, Md: Paul H Brookes Publishing Co; 1998

Mason, J. 1995. Cultural competence self-assessment questionnaire: a manual for users. Portland, Ore: Portland State Unviersity.

Morrison, E. 2009 Health care ethics: critical issues for the 21st century. Jones and Bartlett Pub. Sudbury, MA.

Nunez, A. Transforming cultural competence into cross-cultural efficacy in women's health education. A*cad Med.* 2000;75:1071-1080.

Pope-Davis, D., Eliason, M. Ottavi, T 1993. Exploring multicultural competencies of occupational therapists: Implications for education and training. J of Occupational Therapy, 47, 838-844.

Pope-Davis, D., Ottavi, T 1994. Examining the association between self-reported multicultural counseling competencies and demongraphic variables among counselors. J Couns Dev. 72:651-654.

Purnell, L., Palunka, adapted from Purnell, L. The Purnell Model for C C. In: Purnell L., Palunka, B. eds. . Transcultural health care: A culturally competent approach. 2nd ed. – p.10 F. A. Davis. Phila. 2003 pp8-40.)

Purtilo, RB. Thirty-First Mary McMillan Lecture: A time to harvest, a time to sow: ethics for a shifting landscape. *Phys Ther.* 2000;80:1112-1119.

Ravaud, JF, Stiker, HJ 2001 *Inclusion/exclusion: An analysis of historical and cultural meanings.* In: eds. Albrecht, Selman, and Bury Handbook of disability studies. Thousand Oaks, CA. Sage Pub. Pp.490-512.

Schim, S., Doorenbos, A., Benkert R., Miller J. Culturally *Congruent Care: Putting the Puzzle Together . J of Transcultural Nursing.* April 2007; Vol. 18, No. 2 pp 103-110.

Schim, S., Doorenbos, A., Miller J., Benkert R. (2003) *Development of a cultural competence assessment instrument. J of Nursing Measurement,* Vol.11, no. 1, spring/summer 2003, pp29-40.

Smith, L. 2001. Evaluation of an educational intervention to increase cultural competence among registered nurses. J Cult Diversity. 2001;8(2): 50-63.

Sodowsky, G. Taffe, R. Gutkin T, Wise S. 1994. Development and applications of the multicultural counseling inventory: a self-report measure of multicultural competencies. J Couns Psych. 1994;41:137-148.

Stuart, MR, Lieberman JA 3d, eds. The fifteen minute hour: applied psychotherapy for the primary care physician. 2d ed. Westport, Conn.: Praeger, 1993:101-83.

Tervalon, M. & Murray-Garcia, 1998. Cultural humility versus cultural competence: A critical distinction in defining physician training outcomes in multicultural education. J of Health Care of Poor and Underserved. 9 (2), 17-125.

Tervo, R, Azuma S, Palmer G, Redinius P 2002 *Medical students'attitudes toward persons with disability: a comparative study.* Archives of Physical Medicine and Rehabilitation 83(11):1537-42.

Tylor, E. B. (1958) Primitive culture. New York: Torchbooks. (Original work published in 1871)

Westbrook, M, Legge V, Pennay M 1993 *Attitudes towards disabilities in a multicultural society.* Social Science and Medicine Vol.34 no.5:615-623.

Section III: Disability and Culture: An International Perspective

Chapter 11: The Nature of Disability in the United Kingdom and Multi-cultural influences

Patricia Smith

Introduction

In this chapter, I will look at the notion of disability in the United Kingdom (UK), highlighting issue around independent living, and accessibility to services particularly for ethnic minority groups in the UK, social change and attitudes to disability. Most importantly, I will address some of the legislative changes on disability in the UK and the impact on those living with disability in the United Kingdom.

The Culture of Living with Disability in the UK

The Equality Act (2010) defines a disabled person as one who has a physical or mental impairment that has a substantial and long term adverse effect on his or her ability to carry out day-to-day activities. These impairments may include, loss of limbs, multiple sclerosis, heart disease, Down's Syndrome, learning difficulties, mental health problems such as depression and anxiety. In the UK, people living with disability expect greater help from the government in caring for their family members who experience living with a disability (Hitchcock et al, 1998). As such, there has, in British culture been a tradition of lobbying for legislative and parliamentary involvement around issues of disability (Hitchcock et.al, 1998, Parrrish & Kay, 1998, Richardson, 1997). In the UK, the concept of disability has moved from being seen as a personal tragedy to one of social and environmental barriers in society. These and other models have been discussed in detail in chapter 2.

In spite of the acknowledgment of the need for government support for people living with disability, statistics have shown that there is a disparate between what is expected and what in reality is happening for those living with disability. For example, according to the statistics put forward by the Family Resources Survey (2010-2011) there are over eleven million people with a limiting long term illness, impairment or disability in Great Britain. Many of these individuals suffer long-term pain and have severe difficulties in moving around. In the UK, the most commonly-reported impairments are those that affect mobility, lifting and carrying (Family Resources Survey, 2010-20110). The prevalence of disability rises with age with around 6 per cent of children being disabled compared to 15 per cent of working age adults and 45 per cent of adults over State Pension age in Great Britain (Family Resources survey, 2010-2011). Further, the Equality and Human Rights Commission (2009) has stated that 58% of people over 50 years will have a long term health condition by 2020. This is significant in the UK because this highlights the needs for changes within the NHS which focuses on Patient Centred Practice and includes those with disabilities (NHS business Plan, 2013; Toms & Harrison, 2002). There needs to be options for people to be able to manage long-term health care problems.

However, over a quarter of disabled people say that they do not frequently have choice and control over their daily lives (ONS, 2011) and that disabled people are significantly more likely to experience unfair treatment at work than non-disabled people. In 2008, nineteen per cent of disabled people experienced unfair treatment at work compared to 13 per cent of non-disabled people. Disabled people were more likely to report unfair treatment and discrimination (Fevre, 2008). Around a third of disabled people experience difficulties related to their impairment in accessing public, commercial and leisure goods and services (ONS, 2010). In addition, people living with disability remain less likely to participate in cultural leisure and sporting activities than non-disabled people (ONS, 2011).

These statistics highlight the fact that in spite of the attempts by government to address disability issues through legislative changes around disability, there are still difficulties that people living with disability experience in their everyday lives. One body that plays an integral part in addressing some of these life experiences is the National Centre for independent Living and the Disabled living Foundation.

Independent Living

As the awareness of disability grows the term "disability" should not be equated with "inability" and advocates for disability rights see that there is a sense of empowerment in the term, especially for those living with disability that experience similar situations of social exclusion, discrimination and unemployment (Disability Discrimination Act, 1995). Living with a disability presents many challenges and in the UK, there is a culture of independent living for persons who experience disability. For most people living with a disability in the UK, there are opportunities for creativity in their quest for independent living.

Independent living is about disabled people having the same level of choice, control and freedom in their daily lives as any other person. Many people with disability want to be able to make choices about how they live. People living with disability want to lead an independent life as much as possible. Living a more independent life does not mean that people experiencing disability should not get support from social services. Neither does it mean that the carers and families are not important in the lives of disabled people. Instead, it means that with support from the social services, people living with disability are given the opportunity to make choices about how they would like to live their lives and to do so as independently as possible.

For instance the National Centre for independent Living and the Disabled living Foundation advocate the Independent Living Strategy. The Independent Living Strategy (ILS), published in March 2008, sets out actions aimed at improving the choice and control disabled people have over the services they need to live their daily lives. The aims of the strategy are that:

1. Disabled people (including older disabled people) who need support to go about their daily lives will have greater choice and control over how support is provided
2. Disabled people (including older disabled people) will have greater access to housing, education, employment, leisure and transport opportunities and to participation in family and community life.

This is supported by the Independent Living Scrutiny Group (ILSG) which is an independent group of disabled people. They give their views on how the ILS should progress and advises the government on the progress of the delivery of the ILS. This is an important part of the process and it is in keeping with the Hospital and Community Health Service (HCHS) agenda for change which talks about the patient's choice in accordance with the NHS plan (DOH, 2000:3). One of the main findings that came out of the report on a review of the ILSG was that disabled people felt that there was a large gap between national policy aims and local implementation and that this bridge between rhetoric and reality should be closed (ILSG, 2009).

In addition, there is the Independent Living Review project team which works in partnership with disabled people, making sure that the people whose lives are affected by policies have had a chance to influence and shape the project. In developing the Independent Living Strategy the project team also worked with government departments.

However, in spite of the work of the National Centre for independent Living and the Disabled living Foundation, there are several issues such as transport and mobility, accessibility to the NHS, disability benefits and costs, employment and communication which needs to be addressed and will be discussed below:

Transport and Mobility

In order to maintain an independent lifestyle disabled people in the UK see the need to having good accessible transport that allows good links to work, community involvement, and prevents isolations (ILGS, 2001). These changes have become evident in some areas of public transport e.g. some buses and trains. However alongside this is the need for a greater understanding and involvement of non-disabled people in promoting a more positive personal attitude towards those living with disability and to eliminate stigmatization and discrimination towards disabled people. For instance, non-disabled people need to be more cognizant of the concept of space around those with disabilities and be willing and allow the space needed for those with disability to access public transports or public buildings with ease and comfort or without bringing undue attention to any 'differences' which can be seen as a patronising.

In a document published by the Department for Transport and Disabled Persons Transport Advisory Committee in 2012, it was reported that transport should be easy for everyone to use. Making sure that access to buses, coaches, trains and taxis is hassle-free for all will reduce the number of car journeys and therefore help to reduce carbon emissions (Policy Gov. UK, 2012; Department for Transportand Transport Scotland, 2010). It stipulated that all transport, buses, trains and coaches should be easily accessible for all disabled people including wheelchair users. This is supported by the Equality Act (2010) which is the product of amendments to the Blue Badge scheme (1971) which was developed as part of the Chronically Sick and Disabled Persons Act (1970).

While there have been steps made in the UK to address disability and transport, more needs to be done and the railway system is still working to make trains more accessible for those living with disability by expanding and improving the rail network system (Department for Transport Policy document, 2006).

Closely linked to the transport system is the accessibly of people with disability accessing health & social services. This is so because many disabled people need to use public transportation to get to hospitals, clinics and social services.

Accessibility to the National Health Service (NHS) & Social Service

People living with disability in the UK have many wide and varied experiences of access to the NHS services. For example, some of the challenges around accessibility to the NHS for children with disabilities are centred on issues around 'flexibility', 'parking', the physical space including the waiting areas and consultant's rooms and last but not lease, health professionals understanding and knowledge of disabilities and communication (Wharton, et al, 2005). This is supported in other research (Alborz, 2005) which has also highlighted the lack of interpersonal skills and lack of communication as barriers to the uptake of health care services for people with learning disabilities. However, the underlying legislative force behind these issues is the Disability Discrimination Act (1995) which gives disabled people important rights of access to health services and social services, such as doctors' surgeries, dental surgeries, hospitals and mobile screening units. In this Act disabled people also have a right to information about healthcare and social services in a format that is accessible to them (Disability Discrimination Act (1995). Accessibility includes things such as large print literature, braille of the visually impaired and interpreters for the hearing impaired.

In recent times, the Disability Discrimination Act (1995) has been extended and developed into the Disability Discrimination (NI) Order (2006) which gives people with disabilities rights in the areas of, employment, education, access to goods, facilities and services, including larger private clubs and transport services, buying or renting land or property, including making it easier for people with disabilities to rent property and for tenants to make disability-related adaptations (Disability Discrimination (NI) Order 2006).

The recent New Equality Act (2010), also attempts to address these issues. This is highlighted in the statements from reports such as"the duty to make reasonable adjustments to remove barriers for disabled people" or "the duty to make reasonable adjustments aims to make sure that a disabled person can use a service as close as it is reasonably possible to get to the standard usually offered to non-disabled people" (New Equality Act, 2010). The duty should be 'anticipatory', meaning that a service provider cannot wait until a disabled person wants to use the service. They must think in advance (and on an ongoing basis) about what disabled people with a range of impairments (New Equality Act, 2010).

Disabled people need to use the NHS and social services sometimes to a greater extend than able bodies people. In a Department of Health Policy document (DOH, 2013) efforts have been made to ensure the effective integration of health and social care services for those living with disability. The issue is that in the next 20 years, the percentage of people over 85 will double thus giving rise to more 'complex health needs' especially for those with disabilities so that a combination of services will be needed to address these needs. There is a dilemma around whether people are better treated in hospital or at home and hence the need to have closely joined up services which are properly integrated then the continuity of care needed for the service users, especially for the disabled may become non existent (Health and Social Care Act, 2012). One factor that often gets overlooked is the costs in being disabled.

Disability Benefits and Costs in the UK

Long term conditions and disability carries with it additional costs and in the UK long term disability allowance is put in place to offset some of these additional expenditure (Salway et al, 2007). However, the literature has shown that the accessibility of benefits can vary within different ethnic groups within the UK (Salway, 2007). In this study some of the issues around uptake of benefits amongst different ethnic groups includes lack of knowledge or 'know how' of the system or eligibility for allowances. Some ethnic groups e.g. Bangladeshi and African Caribbean do not want to be labelled or assume the identity of being with a "disabled". As such, this study revealed that a higher percentage of White British people with similar socio-economic status benefited from disability allowance than other Ethnic groups. This points to the need for the UK, a multicultural community to begin to look at ways of improving access to allowances by educating other ethnic groups about their rights and eligibility and how to manoeuvre around the system which is often seen as complex or too stressful for some other ethnic groups.

The need for appropriately sensitive services for those with mental disability is evident for ethnic minority communities (Summers & Jones, 2004) because if the values and beliefs of other religions and cultures are not respected, then this can cause tension for those in need of learning disability services. This brings me to the discussion on disability and unemployment.

Employment

In Srivastava & Chamberlaine (2005), it was found that employers were found to be unresponsive to the needs of workers and had negative attitudes to disability. This is quite alarming in the light of legislation around employment rights and the

Disability Discrimination Act (1995) which states that in all aspects of employment, unless this can be justified, there should be no discrimination around processes including recruitment and selection and all related activities to do with employment such as, work related benefits, references, terms of employment, annual leave, assessments, promotion, pregnancy, maternity and adoption rights, dismissal and redundancy. While these legislations may be in place, there is a need to see how well these are enforced in the work place to to ensure that there is a means for people with disability to be heard and acknowledge in the work place e.g. making reasonable adjustments to the workplace to accommodate those living with disability. This is important as a study by Bell & Heitmueller (2009) has shown that the Disability Discrimination Act (1995) has had no impact on the employment rate of disabled people and may even have possibly worsened it. The study suggests that this may be due to higher uncertainty around litigation costs, lack of awareness about the Disability Discrimination Act (1995) among disabled people and employers, and a lack of financial support. More research is needed in this area. Lastly but by no means least is the question of disability and communication.

Communication

In many instances, people with long term chronic disabilities such as motor neurone disease (MND) in the UK require a multidisciplinary approach to services which depends on establishing good communication pathways between clinicians and service users within a palliative care approach (Hughes et al, 2005). Yet a lack of understanding of the experiences of the lives of these people along with their experiences of the services can pose communication problems. A qualitative study involving semi-structured interviews highlighted these issues (Hughes et al, 2005). It was conducted in three boroughs of London through Kings College hospital. From this study it was recommended that better communication, including service entitlements, improved knowledge were important factors to consider. This had implications for policy makers and professionals in the field.

In a comparative study between Japan and the UK another study, it was found that with increasing severity of disability, there was increasing difficulty in providing services for people living with disability in Southampton, UK (Matsusaka & McLellan, 2003). This again highlights the need for better communication within the MDT networks.

Conclusion

The culture of disability in the UK is a complex one and whilst there are resources being made available by the government and various institutions to address the issues, more attention needs to be paid to whether what is written on paper by way of government Acts and Policy is the actual reality in the lives of those with disabilities. Some parts of Britain are highly multi-cultural and therefore there are different layers to the understanding of culture of disability in the UK. Embedded in the complexity of providing accessible health care services, housing, employment, transportation, leisure and social amenities so that people living with disability can be as independent as possible, there is the potential that ethnic and racial discrimination can complicate the issues even further. A lot more work needs to be done to help people living with disability in the UK achieve their goals and attain an independent life as much as possible.

References

Alborz, A; McNally, R; Gleninning, C (2005) Access to health care for people with learning difficulties in the UK: mapping the issues and reviewing the evidence. J Health Serv Res Policy 10 (3) 173-82.

Curtis, J (2003) Employment and disability in the united Kingdom: and outline fon recent legislative and policy changes. Work 20 (1) 45-51.m

Department for Transport and Transport Scotland (2010) Accessible train station design for disabled people: A code of practice. A joint publication by Department for Transport and Transport Scotland.

Department for Transport policy document (2006): Railways for all Strategy.

Department of Health policy Document (2013): Making sure Health and Social Care services work together.

Health and Social Care Act, 2012).

DOH Rights of Access to Health and Social Care
http://www.nidirect.gov.uk/index/information-and-services/people-with-disabilities/everyday-life-and-leisure/everyday-access/access-to-everyday-services.htm

DOH (2006) Disability Discrimination (NI) Order.
http://www.nidirect.gov.uk/disabled-peoples-rights-in-everyday-life

DOH (1995) Disability Discrimination Act http://www.nidirect.gov.uk/disabled-peoples-rights-in-everyday-life

DOH (1995) http://www.nidirect.gov.uk/index/information-and-services/people-with-disabilities/employment-support/your-employment-rights/employment-rights-and-the-disability-discrimination-act.htm

Family Resources Survey (2010-2011)

Fevre, R; Nichols, T; Prior, G; Rutherford I (2008) The Fair Treatment at Work: Findings from the 2008 survey. Employment relations Research Series No. 103.

Gaskell, S; Nightingale, S (2010) supporting People with Learning Disabilities in Acute Care. Nurs Stand Jan- 6-12. 24 (18) 42-48.

Hitchock, R; Hutchings, C. J; Stephenson, S; Ward, C. D (1998) neurological rehabilitation in Indonesia and the UK: differences and similarities. J Allied health 27 (1) 45-9

Hughes, R. A; Sinha, A; Higginson. I; Down,K; Leigh, P. N (2005) Living with Motor neurones diseases: lives experiences of service and suggestions.

Independent living Scrutiny Group Annual Report (2009) -

J Health Econ. 2009 Mar;28(2):465-80. doi: 10.1016/j.jhealeco.2008.10.006. Epub 2008 Nov 5. The Disability Discrimination Act in the UK: helping or hindering employment among the disabled?Bell D1, Heitmueller A.

Matsusaka, N; McLellan, D. L (2003) Experiences of professionals providing community care for disabled people in Nagasaki and Southampton

NHS Plan (2013) - Putting Patient First: The NHS England Business Plan for 2013/14 - 15/16). NHS England. J Rehabil med (42 Suppl) 4-24.

Office for National Statistics Opinions Survey((2011) Initial Investigation into subject well-Being form the Opinions survey.

Office for National Statistics Opinions Survey((2011) Taking Part survey. Department for culture, media and sport.

Parrish. A; Kay, B (1998) Exploring NHS executive document signposts for Success. Br. J Nurs 13;7 (8) 478-80.

Richardson, M (1997) Addressing barriers: disable rights and the implication for nursing of the social construct of disability J Adv Nurs. 25 (6) 1269-75.

Salway, S; Platt, L; harriss, K; Chowbey, P (2007) Long-term health conditions and Disability Living Allowance: exploring ethnic differences and similarities in access. Social Health Illn.29 (6) 907-30.

Srivastava, S; chamberlain, A (2005) Factors determining job retention and return to work for disabled employees: a questionnaire study of opinions of disabled people's organization in the UK. J rehabil. Med 37 (1) 17-22.

Summers S. J; Jones J (2004) Cross-cultural working in community learning disabilities services: clinical issues, dilemmas and tensions. J Intellect Res 48 (Pt 7) 687-94.

for change. Health Soc Care community 13 (1) 64-74.

Toms, J and Harrison, K (2002) 'Living with Chronic Lung Disease and the effect of Pulmonary Rehabilitation - Patient's perspective' *Physiotherapy,* 88 (10) pp 605-619.

Wharton, S; Harmes, A; Milner, H (2005) the Accessibility of General NHS services for children with disabilities. Child Health Care Dev. 31(3) 275-82.

Chapter 12: The Nature of Disability in South Africa and the Role of Primary Health Care

T. Puckree and T. Nadasan

"The grant is what I eat (MacGregor, 2006)", is not a realistic view of disability in South Africa, but is a contributory factor. In this country disability is real but it is clouded by other realities such asthe harshness of living in post apartheid South Africa, the varied cultural and traditional beliefs, challenges of living in rural and remote areas, and the lack of child care facilities for low income households where the need to work overrides homecare for disabled individuals. The latter is colored by the reality of a social grant being equal to more than half of a full time salary (Mac Gregor, 2006).

The economic struggles of the unskilled and unemployed people of South Africa may be reflected as a negotiation of disability grant allocation in a local setting. The stresses associated with coping in a harsh environment leads to a condition called "having nerves". A community based doctor within the primary health care system must make this diagnosis which is often sufficient to access a disability grant (Macgregor, 2006). The ability to access a disability grant may contribute to inflating the overall prevalence of disabled people in the country. The widening gap between rich and poor South Africans makes the disability grant and old age pensions the only hope of income for many people living in townships like Khayelitsha, an urban township in Cape Town.

Traditional healers are a recognized part of the health care system as discussed in previous chapters. From a cultural and traditional perspective, disabled individuals may be managed within this system under the belief that the disability is a product of supernatural powers (Sello et al., 1997, Masasa et al., 2005; Chimhenga and Musarurwa, 2011). Disability is considered taboo and some parents feel ashamed of having a disabled child (Sello et al., 1997). Families manage the associated stigma by isolating the disabled person to the home. The cultural variations, beliefs and attitudes regarding disability are as wide as the ethnic and cultural groups that make up the rainbow nation of South Africa (Masasa et al., 2005). As such the manner in which disability is embraced or stigmatized is informed by these belief systems. Westernized care is only sought when all other attempts to improve the condition fails. Chimhenga and Musarurwa (2011) based on their study in Zimbabwe suggest an integration of traditional healers into the education system in order to tap into indigenous knowledge systems which could eventually erode unhealthy belief systems which affect the lives of disabled people.

Prior to 2009, the South African census statistics (South African Census,1996,2001,2009) defined disability as a physical or mental handicap, which has lasted for six months or more and which prevents the person from carrying out daily activities independently or from participating fully in educational, economic or social activities. The average prevalence rate for disability from 1996 to 2007 obtained through six national surveys was 5.5%. The 1998 prevalence of 5.7% differentiated between urban and rural areas (Schneider et al., 2009). A 0.8% higher prevalence was observed in urban areas. In the wake of the introduction of the ICF, Schnieder et al (2009) reviewed previous estimates of disability in terms of a new measurement instrument. The 2010 General Household survey (GHS), in which disability was defined as a limitation in one or more activities of daily living showed a prevalence of those reporting moderate to severe disability making up a mean of six point three percent (3,3 to 10,1 %) in the nine provinces in South Africa. The Gauteng province recorded the lowest while the highest prevalence was noted in the Free State province. Overall disability prevalence increased by 0.6% (Schneider et. al., 2009).

With legislation supporting them, disabled people have been participating in educational, economic and social activities. Although South Africa does not have a centralized disability legislation, several pieces of legislation and government policy address disability issues eg the Social Assistance Act of 2004, the Employment Equity Act of 1998, and the integrated National Disability strategy of 1997. Duquay (2012) believes that legislation is still based on the medical model of disability rather than a social model which will provide more opportunities for inclusion.

The Strategic Plan for South Africa 2007–2011 (Department of Education, South Africa, 2007) called for the inclusion of persons with disabilities (Shisana et al 2009) into formal structures. Sustained efforts from the Disabled Persons of South Africa (DPSA) has ensured that legislation promoted inclusivity not only at school level, but in higher education, the workplace and the social pension schemes. Equity compliance reports are mandatory and supported by incentives. In addition even though legislation on making the built environment accessible to persons with disability is not enforced, slow progress is made with new buildings complying with minimal requirements to ensure access. The new National Strategic plan (2012-2017) suggests mainstreaming disability considerations into all programmes of government and other sectors in order to address the needs of people with disability in an integrated and coherent manner (Government of South Africa, 2009)

Although the DPSA has been involved in policy regarding HIV prevention in disabled persons, these persons face a real risk of contracting the disease due to their vulnerability to sexual abuse and rape (Rohleder, 2010). The stigma of disability keeps disabled persons homebound in a society where the breadwinners have to go out to work thereby providing opportunities for disabled persons to engage in unsafe sex which exposes them to HIV, AIDS and STI. Vulnerable people like those with disability are affected more by the high crime rate in the country. Rohleder (2010) found that their results support the findings from the international literature that persons with disabilities may be at risk for HIV infection, as a result of engaging in unsafe sex, being vulnerable to sexual abuse and lacking sex education. These individuals then face double discrimination and marginalization (South African National AIDS council, 2008). The South African National Aids council in their 2008 report suggest that a significant proportion of disabled people still face unjust treatment from family, service providers, peers and society as a whole.

The Human Sciences Research Council in South Africa hasreported an HIV prevalence of 14.1% (CI: 9.9– 19.6) among persons who self-reported as having a disability, compared to 10.9% (CI: 10.0–11.9) for the general population (Shisana et al 2009). It is also indicated that in South Africa people living with HIV are not classified as "disabled "even though they can access the disability grant (Hon Bogapane-Zulu, 2009).

Educational Level

Ranchod et al (2009) found that in comparison with the general population, people with disabilities have lower knowledge levels and lack clarity on HIV transmission and prevention. This makes them vulnerable to a range of exposures.

Population Group

From the 2001 census data (Statistics South Africa, 2001), Black Africans have the highest prevalence of "a lot of difficulty" (10.95%) and "unable to do" (2.64%). Indian/Asians have the lowest rate of "some difficulty" (12.27%) and almost the same levels of "a lot of difficulty" (11.20%), suggesting that with this population group a problem is more likely to be seen as resulting in "a lot of difficulty" than in only "some difficulty". The results are, as for gender, complicated by the fact that Africans are historically disadvantaged in South Africa and are therefore poorer and with lower education and less access to health care services. Black Africans make up 79,5% of the total population in South Africa, with Whites, Coloureds and Indians making up 9%, 9% and 2,5%, respectively (StatsSA,2011).

Geographical Location

Schneider et al (2009) used urban and rural classifications as per the 1996 Census in their study. These investigators found that individuals with 'some difficulty' are prevalent in both urban (20.35%) and rural contexts (19.57%). People with "a lot of difficulty" or who are "unable to do" are more likely to be living in rural areas with 15% of rural dwellers reporting these two categories combined compared to only 10% for urban dwellers. This could be attributed to the lack of services in rural areas as well as the reality or perception that the problem is exacerbated by the lack of health and social services. This finding is consistent with that found in the first national survey on disability conducted for the revised WGSS which yields a higher prevalence of disability than the Census 2001viz.

33.24% vs 12.1%, respectively for the population 15 years and older (The South African National Department of Health,1998 (Schneider et al., 1999). The most prevalent difficulties are those for the activities of seeing, walking and climbing steps and remembering. The least prevalent difficulties are for self care and communication. These trends are the same as found in the national disability survey of 1998 (Schneider et al., 1999) and the Census 2001 (StatsSA, 2005).

Socioeconomic Status

Schneider (1999) found that the older, poorer, less educated, unemployed and widowed or divorced respondents reported having difficulties more easily. It was also noted that the disability literature does not show these as established trends compared to that for age. The two National data sets on disability in South Africa (Schneider et al., 1999; StatsSA, 2005) have a similar to prevalence of 5–17% of childhood disabilities, including intellectual disabilities (ID) in children in developing countries around the world (Kromberg et al, 2008). Kromberg et al (2008). In their study in one rural community in South Africa showed that 291 (4.3%) children had at least one of the five disabilities. Intellectual disability occurred in 3.6%, epilepsy in 0.7%, visual disorders in 0.5%, movement disorders in 0.5%, and hearing disorders in 0.3%. More boys than girls with hearing disorders were receiving special education. Many of the affected children were not receiving treatment or education, resulting in a reduction in their quality of life. Traditional healers were attempting to treat epilepsy and seldom referred affected children to hospital, although effective treatment was available there. Genetic factors were involved in about half the conditions, but genetic services were negligible

Haywood (2004) noted that the prevalence of disability after stroke is similar in South Africa to that in more affluent countries, despite the prevalence of stroke itself being two or three times lower than in high-income countries. Hayward (2004) found that in one rural district of one province in SA, Limpopo, the crude prevalence of stroke was 300 per 100 000 people (*Stroke*2004; 35: 627–32).

The move to a hierarchical model of health care with an emphasis on primary health care is not only likely to address the health care needs of persons with activity limitations and restriction of participation but also identify needy individuals so that appropriate interventions can be applied to improve function where applicable. The cooperative relationship between traditional and western medicine will meet the needs of communities holistically and assist in circumventing issues arising out of traditional beliefs and cultural practice. This issue concurs with discussion in previous chapters and continues to be a topic of interest for people working in primary care.

An average African sees disabilities as a punishment for what one has done wrong. Otieno (2009) observed that among the factors contributing to the general apathy and neglect of children with disabilities in Africa are superstitions that regard disability as a curse from the gods. In Africa, to native Africans, the child is an extension of his or her parents' ego and therefore families will regard a disability in a child as a stain in their social status. This accounts for why children with disabilities are sometimes hidden (Abosi., 2007).

The South African Constitution and the Bill of Rights supports the treatment of disabled persons as equal citizens in South Africa (Gathiram 2007; Government of South Africa, 2009). They are entitled to equal opportunities similar to their able bodied citizens. While strategies are in place to improve access to economic and social development of persons with disability and monitoring systems to ensure that their rights are protected, several challenges still remain especially in ensuring that disabled persons can be productive members of the economy. Mashazi (2002) affirmed that the Government of National Unity stood up to the challenge of transforming the health services and accepted the Alma Ata Declaration as a point of departure in readdressing the inequalities and fragmented health services. The government committed itself to transforming the health sector in order to unify the fragmented health services and integrate health personnel at all levels into a comprehensive and integrated national health system.

Van Rensburg (2004) asserts that the underlying philosophy of the restructuring of the health system in South Africa was the Primary Health Care approach. This approach emphasized that a comprehensive promotive, preventive, rehabilitative and curative care provided by the most appropriate PHC facilities was necessary, with priority attention to PHC services in rural and impoverished urban areas. In one of its recommendations, the Truth and Reconciliation Committee (TRC) highlighted the need for redress as far as the provision of PHC was concerned. The Report emphasized the closing of the gap between advantaged and disadvantaged people, thus improving access to health services in an attempt to correct disparities between urban and rural areas.

The KwaZulu Natal Department of Health KZNDOH) developed its five year framework for transformation, in which its vision, mission and core values are explicitly stated (The'Five-Year Framework for Transformation – Increasing Efficiency and Effectiveness: KwaZulu-Natal Department of Health, 1999–2004'). The KZNDOH) aimed to achieve optimal health status for all persons in the Province of KwaZulu-Natal. The mission was to develop a sustainable, coordinated, integrated and comprehensive health system at all levels, based on the primary health care approach through the District Health System (DHS), (KwaZulu-Natal Department of Health, 1999 –2004). The Core values include the following:

- Continual assessment of health and health service needs and priorities to ensure equitable resource allocation through community participation;
- Promote and protect the health of the community and work towards the prevention of disease and injury;
- Ensure access to compassionate and caring health services;
- Promote the provision of comprehensive services that are responsive to the needs of individuals and communities; and
- To deliver high quality, seamless, comprehensive and effective health services in partnership with clients, the public and related agencies in a supportive environment which promotes trust and confidence.

An audit of this seems necessary.

Within the health care system, service delivery takes place at various levels (primary, secondary and tertiary). At all these levels, medical and rehabilitative personnel have to work in collaboration to ensure optimal health care. Thus, the philosophy of a primary health care approach is in keeping with identifying and maximizing quality of life throughpromotion, prevention, treatment/intervention, habilitation and rehabilitation in communities.

CBR is an integral part of PHC and its principles are applicable at all levels of service delivery, from community to tertiary level. As a strategy within community development for the rehabilitation, equalization of opportunities and social integration of people with disabilities it is implemented through the combined efforts of disabled people themselves, their families and communities, and the appropriate health, education, vocational and social services (DOH, 2000). CBR ensures the empowerment of people with disabilities, caregivers and parents of disabled children. It is people- centred and driven by focusing on a mutual transfer of skills, knowledge and resources between the community, people with disabilities and service providers (National Rehabilitation Policy, 2000).

In 2001, community service was introduced for all health professionals including newly qualified physiotherapists. This service meant that, upon completion of their University based degrees, graduates were assigned to hospitals where the need for their services was the greatest. A year of compulsory service supported the urgent need for health care in the public sector. Even though it was anticipated that the introduction of community service would alleviate the critical shortage of health care personnel in the public sector, a huge need still exists at the PHC level.

Conclusion

Although many provinces welcomed the additional assistance made available through community service, several challenges associated with placing newly qualified graduates in demanding health care environments needed to be addressed. Transformation in Health Sciences education was identified but its planning and implementation still remains a challenge. Many health care training centres have adopted different strategies to equip their graduates with the required skills but these efforts remain piecemeal and uncoordinated.

Van Rensburg (2004), noted that the PHC and the District Health System (DHS) formed the cornerstones of health reform in South Africa. If successful the PHC approach will ensure an inclusive approach to all living with disability.

References

Abosi, O (2007) The Division for Learning Disabilities of the Council for Exceptional Children Educating Children with Learning Disabilities in Africa. Learning Disabilities Research& Practice, *22*(3), 196–201C _2007

Bogopane-Zulu, HI, South African Parliament, Policy and practice-an example from South Africa in Disability and HIV Policy brief, www.who.int/disabilities/jc1632_policy_brief_disability_en.pdf accessed 10 August 2012

Chimhenga, S, Musarurwa C. 2011) Educating children with special needs in the African context: do teachers and parents subscribe to a common paradigm. Acamemic Research International 1(3): 99-106

Department of Health. HIV and AIDS and STI strategic plan for South Africa, 2007–2011 (Draft 9). Pretoria: Department of Health; 2007. Available from: http://www.doh.gov.za/docs/hivaids-progressrep.html. Access date September 8, 2007.

Department of Health (DOH). 1999. Health Sector Strategic Framework 1999-2004. DOH

Department of Health. July 2001. The District Health System in South Africa: Progress made and next steps. DOH.

DuQuay, P 2010 re-defining disability in South Africa: The social Assistance Amendment bill. http://www.legalfrontiers.ca/2010/04/re-defining-disability-in-south-africa-the-social-assist ... accessed 23 april 2012

Gathiram, N (2008) A critical review of the developmental approach to disability in South Africa. International Journal of social welfare 17(2):146-55. DOI:10.1111/j1468-2397.2007.00551.x

Government of South Africa, Department of Education. 2007 www.education.gov.za/linkClick.aspx?fileticket=6RKGke1%2Fbhi... Accessed 10 August 2012.

Government of South Africa, 2009 www.dwcpd.gov.za/about/strategic_plan/ accessed 10 August 2012

Hayward, P 2004 Stroke disability in South Africa matches more affluent nations LANCET Neurology Vol 3 http://neurology.thelancet.com

Kromberg, J. Zwane, E. Manga, ., Venter, A. Rosen, E. Christianson, A (2008) Intellectual disability in the context of a south African population. Journal of Policy and practice in Intellectual disabilities 5(2):89-95 DOI: 10.1111/j.1741-1130.2008.00153. X

MacGregor, H 'The Grant is what I eat; the politics of social security and disability in the post- apartheid South African State . J. biosoc. Sci. (2006) 38, 43–55, _ 2005 Cambridge University Press.doi:10.1017/S0021932005000957 First published online 3 November 2005

Masasa, T. Irwin-Carruthers S, Faure M (2005) Knowledge of, beliefs about and attitudes to disability: implications for health professionals . South African Family practitioner 47(7):40-44.

Mashazi, M. I. 2002. A model for the integration of provincial and local authority nurses rendering primary health care services in a district. Unpublished Doctoral thesis. University of South Africa.

Otieno, PA (2009) Biblical and Theological perspectives on Disability:Implications on the rights of persons with disability in Kenya. Disability Studies Quarterly 29(4): dsq-sds.org/article/view/988

Ranchod, C. Macdonald C, Schneider M, Swartz L, Braathen S H (2009) HIV/AIDS and sexuality of people with disabilities in South Africa: Are

they at greater risk than non-disabled people?poster presented at AfriNEAD 2009 symposium, Cape Town.
www.afrinead.org/index.php?option=com_content&view=article&id...

Rohleder, P 2010 'They don't know how to defend themselves': Talk about disability andHIV risk in South AfricaDisability and Rehabilitation, 2010; 32(10): 855–863

Schneider, M., Claassens, M., Kimmie, Z., Morgan, R., Naicker, S., Roberts, A., et al. (1999). We also count! The extent of moderate and severe reported disability and the nature of the disability experience in South Africa. Study undertaken for the national Department of Health, Pretoria. CASE. Available at http://www.doh.gov.za/facts/index.html.

Schneider, M, Dasappa P, Neloufar Khan N, Azam Khan A (2009) Measuring disability in censuses: The case of South Africa ALTER, European Journal of Disability Research 3: 245–265

Sello, TM, Levitz A, Kemper GD (1997) The attitudes of Xhosa parents towards the education of cerebral palsied children. Educare 26(1,2): 68-75.

Shisana, O, Rehle T, Simbayi LC, Zuma K, Jooste S, Pillayvan-Wyk V, Mbelle N, Van Zyl J, Parker W, Zungu NP, Pezi S, 2009 the SABSSM III Implementation Team. South African national HIV prevalence, incidence, behaviour and communication survey 2008: a turning tide among teenagers?. Cape Town: HSRC Press; 2009.population

South African National AIDS council, 2008 HIV,AIDS and Disability in South Africawww.dcdd.nl/data/1247130050619_Report%20-%20HIV%20AIDS.. Accessed 10 August 2012

StatsSA (2005). Census 2001: prevalence of disability in South Africa. Report No. 03-02-44. Statistics South Africa: Pretoria.

Statistics South Africa.www.southafrica.inf/about/people/population.htm accessed 10 August 2012

Van Rensburg, H. C. J. 2004. Health and Health Care in South Africa. 1st edition. Pretoria: J. L Van Schaik Publishers.

World Health Organization. (1985). Mental Retardation: meeting the challenge. Joint Commission on International Aspects of Mental Retardation. WHO offset publication No 86. Geneva

Chapter 13: Attitudes on Disability in China and the Influence of Traditional Chinese Medicine

Weisi Song

The issue of disability is nothing new in Chinese culture. Several disabling conditions were recorded in ancient Chinese historical classics, like Shiji and Hanshu. The cultural attitudes of Chinese people towards disability are best viewed through its three main religions or philosophies: Confucianism, Buddhism and Daoism.

Confucianism was founded by Kong Fuzi (551B.C—449B.C) about 2500 years ago. Its core principle is to be kind and respectful to others, whether they are rich or poor, healthy or ill. In treating disabled people, it stressed that all disabled people should be treated equally, "treat the elderly disabled people as if they were your parents or grandparents; treat the disabled children as if they were your children or grand children". There is no way that anyone can be treated differently because of their disability. It was said the Kong fuzi had 72 students, who were all famous scholars. Some of these scholars were disabled. Kong Fuzi treated them the same as other able bodied students.

Buddhism originated from India and was introduced to China in the late Han Dynasty (206B.C.-220A.D.) Its core principle is yin guo bao ying, which means your daily life and activities will affect your later life or after life. Buddhism encourages people to behave in a manner that does no harm to any other living thing. Of particular importance was the attention paid to sympathy and tolerance. With regards to disability, Buddhism suggested that the public should show great sympathy and support to disabled people and try to create a comfortable and friendly environment for them. There would therefore be hope for the disabled. The lives and conditions of disabled people are further improved by praying to Buddha and by doing good deeds in society. According to some Buddhist stories, it is not uncommon for those who used to be blind or deaf to now be able to see and hear again after doing good deeds or after getting involved with charity.

Daoism has a more positive approach towards disability. Its main philosophy is balance and harmony (Jung, 1989). It stresses that everything in the universe has two sides: yin and yang or negative and positive polarities. Under certain circumstances, yin and yang will transform into each other (Huang & Maoshing, 1995). This principle can also be applied to disability. In Chinese culture, disability is seen as an unfortunate experience but once it has occurred Chinese culture dictates that there is no point in being upset about it. The person who is affected by a disability would be encouraged to change it into a positive experience. As one of the Chinese poet Li Bai said:

"Since I was born in this world, I must be of some use to it".

Daoism encourages disabled people to pursue the positive side of life. For example, those who were born blind normally have an extremely good sense of hearing and are very good with their hands; they are encouraged to get involved with musical study or Chinese Tuina massage (acupressure). In this way they will not only learn some skills, but also give something back to the society, which in turn gives them a sense of great pride and confidence. Actually some of China's best acupressure practitioners are blind people, who can treat various illnesses from muscular-skeletal complaints to internal problems.

Music is another area that blind people have made a great contribution. Hua Yanjun for example, was born blind and showed a great interest in music when he was young. Luckily his parents discovered his gift for music and sent him to a famous local musician. He made such great progress in music study that he composed" Er quan ying yue" (moon in two streams) when he was very young. This music has been very popular ever since and it was voted one of the most popular music in 20 century in China. We can see from the above discussion of the three main religions in China, that it is not difficult to see that Chinese culture encourages a sympathetic, respectable and positive approach to disability, which will be further discussed in the context of Traditional Chinese Medicine (TCM).

Traditional Chinese Medicine, which consists of Chinese herbal medicine, acupuncture, tuina (Chinese massage), qigong (breathing exercise) and food therapy, is a very important part of Chinese culture and philosophy. It has been applied in China for over 5,000 years. Its theory is based on Chinese culture and years of living and working experience of generations of Chinese people. It also has strong link with the three major religions mentioned above, especially Daoism. Its main theories are yin and yang theory and qi and blood theory.

Yin and Yang Theory

The yin and yang states that there are two fundamental principles or forces in the universe supplementing and opposing each other. Forces that are active, warm, bright are *yang* in nature while those that are still, cold and dark are *yin* in nature. When yin and yang are in balance, the human body is healthy and free of illness; when yin and yang are out of balance, many kinds of illness, including disability, will arise.

Qi and Blood Theory

It is not difficult to understand the notion and function of blood. As for qi, it is a unique term in TCM. Qi means the fundamental substance that comprises the body and provide vital energy for the activities of the body. It consists of three parts: qi from the parents (in born qi), qi from the air (kong qi) and qi from water and food (grain qi). It is essential for the qi and blood to run smoothly in the body, nourishing different organs internally and skin, muscles and joints externally. Deficiency of qi and blood, as well as stagnation of qi and blood, can be a major cause of many illnesses, including disability.

Based on the yin and yang and qi and blood theory, an analysis of imbalances in TCM helps the practitioner to determine the cause of illness and develop an appropriate treatment plan.

Causes of Disability in TCM

There are numerous causes of disability and in Chinese culture they have been identified as described below:

Inborn Disability

This refers to people who are born with a disability. In TCM it is understood that the following factors can affect the inborn qi of the baby, thus causing disability.

Life style of parents: In TCM, the life style of the parents, especially the mother, plays an important role in the health of a baby. If the parent lives an unhealthy lifestyle, such as drinking, smoking, overindulgence in certain foods, lack of sleep and poor nourishment, this will affect the inborn qi of a baby, leading to disability related diseases.

Emotional status of the parents, especially the mother. Practitioners of TCM and conventional medicine have realized that happy motherhood is essential for the baby's growth and development. Long term emotional stress in the mother can affect the baby severely, which could lead to disability. For example, if the mother keeps getting angry constantly during her pregnancy, it will affect the liver function of the baby, possibly leading to the baby being born blind; if the mother lives in fear during the pregnancy, it will affect the function of the baby's kidney, subsequently affecting the growth and development of the baby, including hearing loss and deaf in certain cases.

Time for conceiving: In TCM the belief is that human beings are part of nature and human activities, including conception and should therefore follow the cycles of nature. According to TCM, the best time to conceive is in early spring, which is the time for sowing seeds in the field and the time when things begin to grow in nature. It is strongly advised not to conceive when the weather is unstable or extreme, for example, when there is thunder, heavy rains, strong wind or earth quakes, as these kinds of weathers can affect the baby's inborn qi.

Acquired Disability

In addition to inborn disability, Chinese people also belief that one can acquire a disability through many factors and these are summarized as follows:

Life style: This is a major causative factor in disability. For example, an unhealthy diet, lack of exercise and long term emotional stress are some of the main causes of stroke. In TCM culture, the above factors can affect the smooth flow of qi and blood in the body, disturb the balance of the yin and yang thereby leading to signs and symptoms such as paralyze, dizziness and speech loss.

Casualties from wars and conflicts: Throughout history, China has been invaded by Mongolians and other tribes on many occasions. There were always severe wars and conflicts before dynasties changed and all of these were major causes for war casualties including disability.

Accident and occupation related injuries: Nowadays, accidents and occupationally related injuries such as serious car accidents, falling from high buildings, electric shocks, are some of the main causes of disability. These affect the smooth flow of qi and blood, damages muscles, ligaments, bones and joints externally and also the brain and other major organs internally.

Natural disaster: In China, natural disasters are mainly earth quakes. Due to the nature of earthquakes, which are very difficult to predict as it happens abruptly, it is quite common for the survivors of earthquake to suffer from broken bones, internal organs failure as well as emotional trauma. The physical suffering and emotional trauma after an earthquake can affect the yin and yang balance of the body, affecting the flow of qi and blood, thus causing numerous kinds of ailments which can lead to various types of disabilities.

Overall it is believed all the above factors may affect the harmonious balance of yin and yang of the body, retard the free flow of qi and blood, thereby causing illnesses and disability.

It is not easy to discuss the treatment of disability by TCM in this short chapter. I will therefore outline the treatment of stroke by using TCM as an example. Hopefully, this will provide an insight into treatment principles of TCM. Through years of studies and practice, the TCM practitioners would have built up an abundance of effective methods in treating signs and symptoms caused by stroke.

The Main Signs and Symptoms after Stroke

*Facial hemiparalysis*is one of the main signs of a stroke and this can give rise to retarded speech and hemiplegia. TCM treatment for stroke include: acupuncture, acupressure, Chinese herbal medicine, qigong and food therapy.

In the early stages of a stroke, acupuncture needles are applied to selected points to improve qi and blood flow to the affected area, including the affected brain tissues, in order to build up muscle strength in the extremities as well as to reduce the anxiety and stress levels of the patients.

In combination with acupuncture, Chinese massage is also applied to strengthen the effects of acupuncture. It can be applied on a daily basis to the patient in order to build up muscle strength, to improve blood circulation and to lubricate the joints.

Chinese herbal medicine also plays a very important role in the treatment of stroke. Different herbs are prescribed to the patient according to the pattern identification of the stroke to help to re-balance the yin and yang of the body. Herbs can also be applied to treat stroke related illness, like lung infection, urinary infection, constipation and bed sores.

Besides, food therapy plays an important role in TCM. There is a saying in Chinese culture which goes:

> "Those who can treat their patients with foods only are the best doctors in the world".

Food not only provides energy and the material base for normal human activity, it can also be used for the prevention and treatment of various diseases. In the treatment of stroke using a TCM approach, the patient should avoid heavy, greasy, salty and sugary food and drink. Instead they should adopt a'five colour foods' approach in their menu, these colours being: red, yellow, white, green and black. Red relates to foods such as tomatoes and pomegranates. Yellow foods include carrots, oranges and pumpkins. White foods are rice, oats and sweet potatoes Green foods are fruits and vegetables such as kiwi, celery and Chinese leaves to name a few. Green also includes green tea. Black means black mushroom, especially the one called 'wood ear'. All the foods mentioned above should help improve qi and blood flow, prevent reoccurrence of stroke.

The importance of the patient getting involved in the treatment of their stroke is stressed by the TCM practitioner. Patients are encouraged to keep a positive mind, to be kept away from stressful and depressive situation. They are also encouraged to do qigong and taichi exercise, like eight section brocade, through a combination of slow deep breathing techniques, smooth stretching of the body, with a focused and concentrated mind in order to enhance the free flow of qi and blood and increase the mobility of the affected limbs.

Generally speaking TCM plays a positive role for people with disabilities. It is worth mentioning that many TCM practitioners are disabled themselves. Because they are disabled, they fully understand the difficulties and hardship facing their counterpart and patients. They work very hard in the TCM field and have made great contribution to the well being of the society. For example, Mr Huang Fumi (215-282) suffered from stroke and serious arthritis when he was young. Through self studying acupuncture, he not only cured himself but also treated hundreds of patients from his region. He compiled the famous book, zhenjiu jia yi jing, A-B Classic of Acupuncture and Moxibustion, which is the first acupuncture classic in Chinese history. Another example is Tuina practitioners. Many Tuina practitioners in China are blind. Though they cannot see, they have very sensitive hands and are very good at various manipulative massage techniques. In Beijing there is a Tuina hospital where most of the doctors are blind or partially sighted. They treat hundreds of patients on a daily basis and also teach students from overseas.

It is estimated that the population of disabled people in China is 6,000,000, which is about 4.6 % of the total population. They are encouraged to get involved in social activities and develop their potentials to their fullest. This is not only the aim of the government, but also the responsibility of each individual in China. TCM practitioners have a great role to play in helping disabled people in China realize this potential.

I will now outline a case study which applies some of the principles that I have discussed.

Case Study

Name: Mr Wong Age: 62 Occupation: accountant

Main complaint: stroke 6 weeks.

Medical history

Previous history: The patient has suffered from high blood pressure and diabetes for about six years. Even though he was prescribed Western medicine by his GP to control his blood pressure, he did not take them regularly and subsequently his blood pressure was not well controlled. Six (6) weeks ago, while he was watching TV, he complained of a distending headache on the left side, dizziness and nausea and then he collapsed and lost consciousness. He was rushed to the local hospital and was given a brain MRI scan, the result of which was a cerebral infarction (left side). After one week of treatment, he regained consciousness, but his speech was unclear and he had difficulty in moving his right arm and leg. He was discharged from the hospital and was waiting for a physiotherapy appointment to help his recovery. He was recommended by some friends to have acupuncture and herbal medicine treatment.

Present Conditions

Asking: Distending headache, mainly on the left side, dizziness, irritable, poor sleep, pain and numbness of the right arms and legs, difficulty with the movement of the right limbs, thirsty, constipation

Listening: His speech was not very clear, but he could answer most questions correctly.

Palpitation: Stiffness and weakness of left arms and legs, no signs of swelling and water retention. Weak and thin pulse.

Observing: Slightly overweight, flushed face. Deviation of mouth towards right. Tip of the tongue points towards left while being checked. Red tongue with purple spots and thick and greasy coating.

Western Medical Examination

BP 165/95mmhg, P 80

Left nasolabial groove is shallower than that of left side, tip of the tongue points towards left while being checked, deviation of mouth towards right, the level of muscle strength of left arm and leg: 0. Hypotonus left arm and leg. Pain sensation also reduced on the left side. Tendon reflex of left side: overactive Barbinski sign left(+), right(+)

TCM diagnosis: Stroke (Upward of liver yang and qi and blood stagnation)

Western medicine diagnosis: Stroke - cerebral infarction (Cerebrovascular accident - CVA)

Treatment plan: improve blood flow to the affected region, calm down liver yang, improve mobility of the left limbs

Treatment

Acupuncture

Points from the head to increase blood flow to the brain were selected, such as Du 20 and Si Shen Cong; I also selected points near his tongue to improve his speech, e.g lianquan and points from the left arm and leg to improve the muscle strength and mobility and ease the numbness and pain e.g LI11, St36 and GB40.

The acupuncture treatment was applied twice a week to start with.

Food Therapy

The patient was encouraged to avoid heavy, greasy, salty and sugary food. He was advised to follow the five colour food principle, to drink sufficient green tea and to eat good quantities of black mushrooms in order to improve blood circulation and prevent further blood clots in the brain. He was advised to drink a lot of water and to eat water melon everyday to alleviate constipation and prevent urinary tract infection.

Massage

His wife was shown some basic massage techniques to apply on his left arm and leg to improve blood circulation and help to build up muscle strength. His wife was told to apply the massage to him once a day, about 20 minutes for each session.

Herbal Medicine

Bu yang huan wu tang, a classic herbal formula to treat stroke was prescribed to him. It was a very famous and effective formula to treat stroke. It was invented by the renowned TCM practitioner Qingren Wang. The patient was asked to take the formula twice a day.

Results

After five sessions of treatment, the patient showed great improvement. His muscle strength reached level 1 where there was slight movement of his left arm and leg. After another five session's treatment, his muscle strength on the left side reached level 3, speech became much clearer and there was no deviation of the mouth; he was able to carry out some simple daily movement, such as putting on clothes and brushing his teeth. After another 6 weeks of treatment, his left side returned to normal, his speech returned to normal and he returned to work. He was still advised to watch his diet and do some gentle exercise every day, avoid stress and check his blood pressure regularly.

Discussion & Conclusion

This case represents the typical signs of stroke and the diagnosis was confirmed by MRI scan. In this context there may be complementary aspects in Eastern and Western approaches in the diagnosis of disability. However, the theoretical basis of the approach to disability differs culturally in Eastern and Western societies. It should be noted that though the treatment of acupuncture and Chinese herbal medicine offered for this patient might be different from other stroke patients, the principle will be quite similar. Hopefully this case will offer some insight into the treatment of stroke by Traditional Chinese Medicine.

Bibliography & Further Reading

Huang Ti; Maoshing Ni (1995) The Essential text of Chinese Health and Healing: The Yellow Emperor Classic of Medicine: A new Translation of the Neijing Suwen with commentary. Shambala Publications.

Huang-Fu Mi (2005) 4th Edn. The Systematic Classic of Acupuncture and Moxibustion: A translation of the Zhenjiu Jia Yi Jing by Yang Shou Zhong. Blue Poppy Press. A division of Blue Poppy Enterprise Inc.

Jung C. G., Wilhelm R, and Baynes, C. F. (1989) I Ching or Book of Changes (Arkana).

Li Bai: Poems by Li Bai (Li Po)
http://www.goodreads.com/author/quotes/4058. Li_Bai

Chapter 14: Perspectives on Disability in India

Parul Agarwal and G. Arun Maiya

As per the World Health Organization; Disabilityis an umbrella term, covering impairments, activity limitations, and participation restrictions. Impairment is a problem in body function or structure; an activity limitation is a difficulty encountered by an individual in executing a task or action; while a participation restriction is a problem experienced by an individual in involvement in life situations.

"Persons with disabilities include those who have long term physical, mental, intellectual or sensory impairments which in interaction with various barriers may hinder their full and effective participation in society on an equal basis with others." Both these expressions reflect a shift from a medical model to a social model of disability.

Medical Model

In the medical model, individuals with certain physical, intellectual, psychological and mental impairments are taken as disabled. According to this, the disability lies in the individual as it is equated with restrictions of activity with the burden of adjusting with environment through cures, treatment and rehabilitation.

Social Model

In contrast to this, the social model focuses on the society, which imposes undue restrictions on the behavior of persons with impairment. In this, disability does not lie in individuals, but in the interaction between individuals and society. It advocates that persons with disabilities are right holders and are entitled to strive for the removal of institutional, physical, informational and attitudinal barriers in society.

Definition of Disability in the Indian Context

In India, different definitions of disability conditions have been introduced for various purposes, essentially following the medical model and, as such, they have been based on various criteria of ascertaining abnormality or pathologic conditions of persons. In the absence of a conceptual framework based on the social model in the Indian context, no standardization for evaluating disability across methods has been achieved. In common, different terms such as disabled, handicapped, crippled, physically challenged, are used inter-changeably, indicating noticeably the emphasis on pathologic conditions.

Sources of Disability Statistics in India

In any society estimation of the population suffering from physical or mental infirmities, with reasonable accuracy, is a challenging task. In the absence of a complete and perfect administrative statistics, recourse is taken through surveys and censuses in spite of their inherent limitations in netting rare personal characteristics. The Persons with Disabilities (Equal Opportunities, protection of Rights and Full Participation) Act which came into force in 1995, imposes specific obligation on the government to undertake surveys, investigation and research concerning causes of disability.

In India, the major sources of statistics on disability are the decadal Population Censuses and the regular large scale sample surveys on disability conducted by National Sample Survey Office (NSSO)

Data on the Cause of Disability

The main underlying causes of disability are malnutrition, diseases, congenital factors, accidents and violence, inadequate hygiene, landmine explosions, lack of access to a health care system, exposure to chemical substances and stresses most of which are preventable.

Issues Related to Disability Policies in India

Discrimination against persons with disabilities, and unwillingness to bear the costs of creating a more accessible environment e.g. at schools or workstations are key obstacles to the improvement of the lives of persons with disabilities.

Poverty is one of the causes of disability. This is because the poor are more exposed to dangerous working and living conditions, including lack of access to healthcare facilities, and poor nutrition, among others. On the other hand, disability can also be a cause of poverty. This is particularly true if the persons with disabilities, and their caretakers, do not have the capacity to generate income for the family. Moreover, there may also be financial constraints brought about by the expensive medical treatment or assistive devices needed by persons with disabilities. Data on income as well as other information regarding the economic status of the household may provide insight into how poverty can affect disability and vice-versa.

Persons with Disability (Equal Opportunities, Protection of Rights and Full Participation) Act 1995

Provision in the Act

The provisions contained in the Persons with Disability (Equal Opportunities, Protection of Rights and Full Participation) Act, 1995, imposes several obligations on the Central and State Governments for taking up various measures to ensure equal participation of people with disabilities in all walks of life. Section 25(a) of the Act specifically mentions that "within the limits of their economic capacity and development, the appropriate Governments and the local authorities, with a view to preventing the occurrence of disabilities, shall undertake investigations and research concerning the cause of occurrence of disabilities". The National Policy for Persons with Disabilities has also recognized that "there is a need for regular collection, compilation and analysis of data relating to socio-economic conditions of persons with disabilities". The Policy has also envisaged that research be undertaken focusing on the following aspects:

- Socio-cultural aspects of disability, which include study of social attitude and behavioral patterns towards persons with disabilities.
- Develop social indicators relating to the education of persons with disabilities in order to analyze the problems involved and take up programs to improve access and opportunities
- Generate statistics about the employment status of persons by type of disability especially for those who become disabled due to accidents and other disasters.
- Study causes of different types and level of incidence of disabilities

The Persons with Disability (PWD) Act (1995) defines disability in terms of extent of impairment of body structure and body function. The context in which the definitions of disability and categories therein are being examined here relates to the classification of person, as disabled or not, by an enumerator who is given a short training in concepts and definitions. Therefore, the definitions under PWD Act need to be converted into definitions, which are simple and tangible from the point of view of the enumerator as well as the respondents

Statistics on Disability in India

Census and NSS surveys are the major two sources of official statistics on disability. But the two differ substantially especially in respect of overall estimates of persons with various types of disability and their age distribution, mainly due to differences in the concepts and definitions as also the data collection methodologies.

The results on disability are available only for census 2001. The census 2011 results on disability are not released up to the time of writing this chapter.

NSS Surveys on Disability

The National Sample Survey made its first attempt to collect information on the number of physically handicapped in its 15th round survey (July 1959-June 1960). NSSO undertook a comprehensive survey on this subject for the first time in the NSS 36th round (July- December 1981) as 1981 was the International Year of the disabled persons. Detailed information relating to magnitude of disability, type of disability, cause, age at onset, type of aid/ appliance used and other socio-economic characteristics was collected in this survey.

At the turn of the new millennium about 21 million people in India were found to have disability as per the official estimate obtained from the Population Census 2001. These included persons with visual, hearing speech, locomotor or mental disabilities, who constituted about 2 percent of the population. On the other hand, NSSO survey on Disability (July – December 2002) also estimated the disabled population in the country as 20.7 million (Table 2 below) along with the variations in definitions (Table 3). Table 4 shows specific data for each disability whileTable 5 shows the distribution of persons with locomotor disability by cause.

Table 2. Figures on Persons with Disabilities based on NSSO 2002 survey (58[th]round) and Census 2001:

Type of disability	NSSO,2002 (lakh)	Census,2001 (lakh)
Locomotor	106.34	61.05
Visual	28.26	106.35
Hearing	30.62	12.62
Speech	21.55	16.41
Mental	20.96	22.64
TOTAL	207.73	219.07

Table 3 - Statement showing the variation in definitions

Category	Census	NSSO	PWD Act
(i)Disability	Five types of disabilities identified for Census 2001	A person with restrictions or lack of abilities to perform an activity in the manner or within the range considered normal for a human being was treated as having disability. It excluded illness/injury of recent origin (morbidity) resulting into temporary loss of ability to see, hear, speak or move.	"Person with disability" means a person suffering from not less than forty per cent of any disability as certified by a medical authority; "Disability" means-(i) Blindness;(ii) Low vision;(iii) Leprosy-cured;(iv) Hearing impairment;(v) Loco motor disability;(vi) Mental illness;(vii) Mental retardation.

Category	Census	NSS	PWD Act
(ii)Mental disability	A person who lacks comprehension appropriate to his/her age will be considered as mentally disabled. This **would not mean** that if a person is not able to comprehend his/her studies appropriate to his /her age and is failing to qualify examination is mentally disabled	Persons who had difficulty in understanding routine instructions, who could not carry out their activities like others of similar age or exhibited behaviours like talking to self, laughing / crying, staring, violence, fear and suspicion without reason were considered as mentally disabled for the purpose of the survey. The "activities like	**"Mental illness"** means any mental disorder other than mental retardation; **"Mental retardation"**means a condition of arrested or incomplete development of mind of a person which is specially characterized by sub normality of intelligence

| | | others of similar age" included activities of communication (speech), self-care (cleaning of teeth, wearing clothes, taking bath, taking food, personal hygiene, etc.), home living (doing some household chores) and social skills. | |

Category	Census	NSS	PWD Act
(iii)Visual disability	A person who cannot see at all (has no perception of light) or has blurred vision even with the help of spectacles will be treated as visually disabled. A person with proper vision only in one eye will also be treated as visually disabled. A person may have blurred vision and had no occasion to test whether his/her eye- sight would improve by using spectacles. Such person would also be treated as visually disabled	By visual disability, it was meant, loss or lack of ability to execute tasks requiring adequate visual acuity. For the survey, visually disabled included (a) those who did not have any light perception - both eyes taken together and (b) those who had light perception but could not correctly count fingers of hand (with spectacles/contact lenses if he/she used spectacles/contact lenses) from a distance of 3 meters (or 10 feet) in good day light with both eyes open. Night	"**Blindness**" refers to a condition where a person suffers from any of the following conditions, namely:- (i) Total absence of sight. or (ii) Visual acuity not exceeding 6160 or 201200 (snellen) in the better eye with correcting lenses; or (iii) Limitation of the field of vision subtending an angle of 20 degree or worse; **"Person with low vision"** means a person with impairment of visual functioning even after treatment or standard refractive

		blindness was not considered as visual disability.	correction but who uses or is potentially capable of using vision for the planning or execution of a task with appropriate assistive device;

Category	Census	NSS	PWD Act
(iv)Hearing disability	A person who cannot hear at all or can hear only loud sound will be considered as having hearing disability. Also a person who cannot hear through one ear but the other is functioning normally is considered as having hearing disability.	This referred to persons' inability to hear properly. Hearing disability was judged taking into consideration the disability of the better ear. In other words, if one ear of a person was normal and the other ear had total hearing loss, then the person was judged as normal in hearing for the purpose of the survey. Hearing disability was judged without taking into consideration the use of hearing aids (i.e., the position for the	**"Hearing impairment"**means loss of sixty decibels or more in the better ear in the conversational range of' frequencies;

		person when hearing aid was not used). Persons with hearing disability might be having different degrees of disability, such as profound, severe or moderate. A person was treated as having 'profound' hearing disability if he/she could not hear at all or could only hear loud sounds, such as, thunder or understands only gestures. A person was treated as having 'severe' hearing disability if he/she could hear only shouted words or could hear only if the speaker was sitting in the front. A person was treated as having 'moderate' hearing disability if his/her disability was neither profound nor severe. Such a person would usually ask to repeat the words spoken by the speaker or would like to see the face of the	

		speaker while he/she spoke or would feel difficulty in conducting conversations.	

Category	Census	NSS
v)Speech disability	A person will be recorded as having speech disability if he/she is dumb. A person whose speech is not understood by a listener of normal comprehension and hearing will be considered having speech disability. A person who stammers but whose speech is comprehensible will not be classified as having speech disability.	This referred to persons' inability to speak properly. Speech of a person was judged to be disordered if the person's speech was not understood by the listener. Persons with speech disability included those who could not speak, spoke only with limited words or those with loss of voice. It also included those whose speech was not understood due to defects in speech, such as stammering, nasal voice, hoarse voice and discordant voice and articulation defects, etc

Category	Census	NSS	PWD Act
vi)Locomotor disability	A person who lacks limbs or is unable to use limbs normally, will be considered having movement disability. Absence of a part of a limb like a finger or a toe will not be considered as disability. However absence of all the fingers or toes or a thumb will make a person disabled by movement. Following persons will also be treated as having movement disability: - If any part of the body is deformed, - Who cannot move himself /herself or without the aid of another person or without the aid of stick etc, - If he/she is unable to move or lift or pick up any small article placed near him. - A person not able to move normally because of problems of joints like arthritis and has to invariably limp while moving	A person with - (a) loss or lack of normal ability to execute distinctive activities associated with the movement of self and objects from place to place and (b) physical deformities, other than those involving the hand or leg or both, regardless of whether the same caused loss or lack of normal movement of body – was considered as disabled with locomotor disability. Thus, persons having locomotor disability included those with (a) loss or absence or inactivity of whole or part of hand or leg or both due to amputation, paralysis, deformity or dysfunction of joints which affected his/her "normal ability to move self or objects" and (b) those with physical	**"Locomotor disability"** means disability of the bones, joints muscles leading to substantial restriction of the movement of the limbs or any form of cerebral palsy. "Cerebral palsy" means a group of non-progressive conditions of a person characterized by abnormal motor control posture resulting from brain insult or injuries occurring in the pre-natal, peri-natal or infant period of development

		deformities in the body (other than limbs), such as, hunch back, deformed spine, etc. Dwarfs and persons with stiff neck of permanent nature who generally did not have difficulty in the normal movement of body and limbs was also treated as disabled.	

Category	PWD Act
(vii)Leprosy cured person	**"Leprosy cured person"** means any person who has been cured of leprosy but is suffering from- (i) Loss of sensation in hands or feet as well as loss of sensation and paresis in the eye and eye-lid but with no manifest deformity; (ii) Manifest deformity and paresis; but having sufficient mobility in their hands and feet to enable them to engage in normal economic activity; (iii) Extreme physical deformity as well as advanced age which prevents him from undertaking any gainful occupation, and the expression "leprosy cured" shall be construed

Table 4: Disability –Specific Data for each disability

Physical Disability	Visual Impairment	Hearing Impairment	Speech Disability	Locomotors Disability	Overlapping
41.32 %	10.32%	8.36%	5.06%	23.04%	11.54%

Table 5: Per 1000 Distribution of Persons with Locomotor Disability by Cause

	Urban	Rural
Paralysis	328	346
Burns	211	25
Cardio-Respiratory diseases	112	115
Old Age	54	49
Cerebral Palsy	48	43
Leprosy	29	41
Polio	30	19
Smoking	20	19
Other illnesses	22	15
Other reasons	146	128

Conclusion

Disability in India is quite prevalent and varied as evidenced by the statistics presented in this chapter. For the most part, disability in India is pathological in nature, occurring due to social, economic and environmental factors mentioned earlier. More standardized methods of evaluating disability in the Indian cultural context are needed and these have to be clearly defined not only from the medical model approach but also from a societal perspective.

References

Census of India (2011); Instruction Manual for Updating of Abridged House-list and Filling up of the Household Schedule

Disability In India (2011) - A Statistical Profile - March 2011

PWD Act, (1995); The Persons With Disabilities: (Equal Opportunities, Protection Of Rights And Full Participation) Act, 1995.

Report No. 485 (58/26/1); NSS 558th round ((July — December 2002)); Disabled Persons in India.

Chapter 15: The Nature of Disability in the Occupied Palestinian Territories (oPt) and the Impact of Working in a Crisis Zone

Lesley Dawson

Introduction

The occupied Palestinian territories comprise the West Bank [including East Jerusalem] and the Gaza Strip (www.wfp.org/occupied-Palestinian-territories). The West Bank is 5,800 sq. km and the Gaza Strip is 365 sq. km, separated by 80 km of Israeli territory (www.fco.gov.uk). The population is estimated to be around 4 million, of whom 50% are refugees and 1.4 million reside in the Gaza Strip (WHO 2009).

This discussion is set within the context of an Arab, mainly Muslim society, with a vocal and educated Christian minority. This Arab world cultural and religious context affects the nature of disability in the oPt. Its values are mainly Muslim and the minority Christian community holds Eastern Christian values, which are closer to Islam than western Christianity (Marsh 2012). In this context the family is more important than the individual, children are very important within the family and it is a patriarchal society with great respect shown to older family members, especially men. While in theory disabled people are accepted in Islamic society (Pervez 2013), physical beauty and wholeness is important for marriage prospects, especially for girls (Sazeims 2013).

The birth of children with disabilities is often seen as a divine punishment and a shame on the whole family, especially the mother and access to rehabilitation for children favours boys more than girls. Disability developed later in life may also be seen as a mark of divine disfavour or testing, unless as a result of an injury sustained in the on-going political conflict (Boston Healing Landscape Project 2012). Those disabled in the political conflict may be viewed as political heroes. Older people disabled as the result of disease will be cared for within the extended family, usually by the women in the family, as is the case in most Arab societies (Al Oraibi et al 2011).

It is not possible to put aside the effects of the political situation when discussing life in the oPt. Occupation, for some residents since 1948, for others since 1967 and refugee status, the effects of the First and Second Intifada [uprisings against Israeli occupation], the setting up of the Palestinian National Authority, the invasion and subsequent closure of Gaza and the bombing of major towns in the West Bank must also be taken into account (Husseini 2007).

The situation in Gaza is particularly problematic with currently 6.5% of the population partly dependant on food aid and 90% of mains water polluted. The economic situation has declined dramatically because the majority of male day workers are unable to exit the area and gain work in Israel. There are limited opportunities for work and a lack of resources with limited access into Gaza of humanitarian aid and other goods (CBM website 2012).

Whether the oPt is part of the developed or the developing world is debatable. Because of their proximity to Israel and social interaction with Israelis, it could be argued that the oPt is part of the developed world and the presence of diseases such as stroke and diabetes would confirm this. However the fact that there is a high incidence of malnutrition, high maternal mortality and child developmental disability points towards them being described as having a developing world status. Some researchers have described Palestinian society as one that is in transition, containing elements of both developing and developed worlds (Bargouthi and Lennock 1997, Dawson 1999, WHO 2009).

The Nature of Disability in the oPt

WHO indicates that 2.5 % of the Palestinian population are affected by disability and 14.8% of the elderly suffer from a disability (WHO 2009). Rehabilitation services are provided by the Palestinian Ministry of Health at national level and Non-Governmental Organisations [NGOs] and the United Nations Works and Relief Association for the Middle East [UNWRA] at intermediate and community levels (Jillson 2001), but much of the long term rehabilitation of those with disabilities is supported by international INGOs (Harami et al 2010).

Palestinian society has concentrated more on physical disability, with sight and hearing impaired people well served with centres in Jerusalem and major towns in the West Bank and Gaza Strip (Jillson 2001), as are children with developmental problems (Bar-Haim et al 2010). As a result of disabilities sustained during the First Intifada, other centres dealing with spinal cord injuries, head injuries and limb gunshot wounds were established, initially by international NGOs which were later transferred to local staff and funding. The model of disability espoused is still mainly a bio-medical one, although the development of Community-Based Rehabilitation [CBR] indicates a move towards a social model of disability (Layton 2009).

Mental disability was much slower to be recognised and provided for. The impetus in this area was provided by depression among male workers unable to gain work, children witnessing confrontations between the Palestinian young male civilians, police and military and the Israeli Defence Force [IDF] and by psychological problems encountered by psychological problems encountered by released prisoners (Giacaman et al 2005).

A lack of provision of facilities has affected the status of disabled people. The number of rehabilitation personnel is similar to Jordan at less than 1 per 10,000 of the population (WHO, 2011:109). The location of rehabilitation centres are in the main conurbations, whilst many of the disabled people live in rural areas with limited transport and problems of movement from area to area, as a result of checkpoints and closures. There are also gender issues, with some clinics maintaining a policy of staff only treating same gender patients.

CBR programmes have had a pronounced impact on the lives of individuals with disability and their families. They have also had a positive impact on awareness, attitudes and practice towards individuals with disability in their communities (Harami et al 2010). However Giacaman (2012) warns that, as this is often provided voluntarily by women in the family, it adds to their already heavy workload in the home.

Developmental disability in oPt may be linked to a range of issues, such as close family marriage leading to congenital problems, poor obstetric services with a lack of sufficient trained midwives and the effects of tear gas on pregnant women. Maternal exposure to psychosocial, economic and political situations is associated with low birth weight (Abusalah and Radwan, 2012) and affects the health of pregnant women and new babies.

Disability sustained as a result of other injuries or disease such as stroke or amputation due to diabetes are quite common (Abu-Rmeilah 2012, Amro 2012). In general, older people are disproportionately represented in disability populations (WHO 2011 page 35) and their disability reflects an accumulation of health risks across a life span (WHO 2011 page 35). However the demographics of disability in the oPt indicate a young population, with around 46% of the population below the age of 15 years of age (WHO 2009 page 3).

Disability as a result of trauma, such as road traffic accidents, gunshot wounds, injuries sustained during shelling, bombing and landmines is seen in Palestinian society (WHO 2011 page 34). Disability is often exacerbated by delays in obtaining emergency health care and rehabilitation. During 2006-2007 during the eruption of the Second Intifada records from three hospitals in Nablus indicate that gunshot wounds were the major cause of head injury (Younis et al 2011). The fact that small towns and villages in the West Bank and Gaza Strip are lacking rehabilitation clinics limits early treatment for traumatic impairments (McCoull 2008). Of the 40,000 Palestinians injured during the political conflict between 2000 - 2003 25,000 were permanently disabled, of whom 500 were children (The Palestinian Monitor 2003). The present political situation would lead one to believe that these statistics will be replicated today.

The Impact of Working in a Crisis Zone

In whatever context, disabled people are those most likely to be undernourished, neglected and at risk in a crisis situation. Violence and humanitarian crises contribute to disability (WHO 2011, Page 59) as discussed in the previous section describing disability caused by trauma. Conflict situations also make people with disabilities more vulnerable (WHO 2011 page 108) as mobility is often limited and they are less likely to be able to evacuate away from violent situations.

There is an obvious impact on patients and their families living outside the main areas of Bethlehem and Ramallah who face long delays at check points and road closures as they seek to gain access to centres of treatment. The inability to access centres in Jerusalem without the appropriate permits and the need to stay in rehabilitation centres causes a dilemma for families with other dependents at home. For Gazans, the near impossibility of gaining permission to leave Gaza (UNOCHA June 2012), the restrictions on travel and the current harsh socioeconomic conditions affect everyone (Jillson 2001).

There is also an impact on healthcare staff who face similar barriers of check points, road closures and lack of transport to access their work settings (UNOCHA September 2011), permits from Israeli authorities and concern about their family whilst the health professional is at work in another location (UNOCHA December 2011). Those living outside the Separation Wall may have to cope with long hours of travel to get to work, the need for permits and the strain of not knowing what will happen from day to day. These restrictions on travel particularly affect women as families may forbid them to travel in conflict situations. All these restrictions contribute to well-trained staff leaving the country because of the political situation.

Conclusion

The nature of disability in the occupied Palestinian territories is a complex issue with many strands. Disability here affects the whole age range, with different causes for childhood and adult disability. Physical disability is better understood than mental disability, although the emergence of psychiatric problems among children and adults as a result of the effects of long-term occupation and political conflict has raised the profile of mental disability. Provision for childhood disability continues to be a priority as does that for those disabled as a direct result of political conflict. Disability resulting from non-political trauma or disease receives limited attention but the increased emphasis on disability in general is beginning to have an impact here.

The impact of the political conflict continues to negatively influence the lives of people with disability, impacts on the development of disability programmes and affects the work and lives of those who provide rehabilitation services for Palestinians with disabilities.

References

Abu-Rmeileh, N. (2012) http//www.thelancet.com/health-in-the-occupied-palestinian-territory-2012)

Abusaleh, A. and Radwan, A. (2012) http//www.thelancet.com/health-in-the-occupied-palestinian-territory-2012)

Al Oraibi, S. Dawson, V. L. Balloch, S. and Moore, A.P. (2011) Impact of culture on rehabilitation services; a Jordanian perspective, International Journal of Disability, Community and Rehabilitation, 8 (1).

Amro, A. (2012) Stroke rehabilitation outcomes for patients in Hebron, Unpublished doctoral thesis, University of Western Cape, South Africa.

Bar –Haim, S. Harries, N. Nammourah. I. Oraibi, S. Malhees, W. Loeppsky J. and Lahat, E. (2010)

Bargouthi, M. and Lennock, J. (1997), Health in Palestine; Potential and challenges. In MAS Discussion Papers, Palestine Economic Research Institute, Jerusalem.

Boston Healing Landscape Project (2001-2012) Islam and Healing: Illness, Boston University School of Medicine, A program for the study of cultural, therapeutic and religious pluralism, www.bu.edu/bhip/Resources/Islam/health/illness html

Christoffen Blinden Mission website (2012) www. cbm.org/Palestine-Gaza_292805.php

Dawson V. L. (1999) Professional development, personality and self-=esteem of Palestinian physical therapists, Chapter 30 in Leavitt, R. L. (Ed) Cross-cultural rehabilitation; an international perspective, W. B. Saunders; Philadelphia

Giacaman, R. Arya, N. and Summerfield, D. (2005) Establishing a mental health system in the Occupied Palestinian Territories, Special paper, *Bulletin of the Board of International Affairs of the Royal College of Psychiatrists*

Giacaman, R. (2012) htttp//www.thelancet.com/health-in-the-occupied-palestinian-territory-2012)

Harami, G. Henley, D. and Greer, C. (2010) Development of a disability programme in the West Bank and Gaza Strip, www.thelancet.com Published online July 2 2010.

Husseini. A. S. (2007) Palestinian refugees in the West Bank and Gaza strip: Health = Development, Medicine and War, Vol 1, Issues 2, 1996.

Jillson, I. (2001a) Caring for the disabled in the West Bank and Gaza, Policy Research incorporated.

Jillson, I. (2001b) List of NGOs working in disability and rehabilitation services in the West bank and Gaza Strip, August 2001

Layton, K. (2009) Paradoxes and paradigms: How can the social model of disability speak to international humanitarian assistance, ANU Undergraduate Research Journal, Vol 1 pages 55-61.

Marsh, L. (2012) Palestinian Christian Theology as a new and contemporary expression of Eastern Christian thought, in Living Stones Yearbook, pages 106-119

McCoull, C. (2008) Occupied Palestinian Territories, *Journal of Mine Action*, Issue 12.1, summer 2008

Palestinian Monitor, Statistics for the Palestinian Intifada, 28 Sept 2000-8 July 2003.

Pervez, S. (2013) Disability in Islam, http:// www.whyislam.org/social-values-in-islam/social ties/disability-in-islam/

Sazeims, (2013) Disabled people get a raw deal in marriage market, http://www.aulia-e-hind.com

World Food Programme www.wfp.org/occupied-Palestinian-territories (accessed 9.1.13)

Younis, R. Younis, M. Hamidi, S. Musmar and Mawson, A. R. (2011) Causes of traumatic brain injury in patients admitted to Rafidia, Al Ittihad and the specialized Arab hospitals. Palestine, 2006-2007, Brain Injury, Vol 25, No 3, pages 282-291.

UNOCHA (2011) Movement and access in the West Bank, United Nations Office for the Co-ordination of Humanitarian Affairs, oPt. September 2011

UNOCHA (2011) East Jerusalem: Key humanitarian Concerns, December 2011

UNOCHA (2012) Five years of blockade: The humanitarian situation in the Gaza Strip, June 2012

UNOCHA (2012), The humanitarian impact of the barrier , July 2012

WHO (2009) Health conditions in the occupied Palestinian territory, including East Jerusalem, and in the occupied Syrian Golan. A62/INF. DOC/2, 14 May 2009, 62nd World Health Assembly.

WHO (2011) World Report on Disability, World Health Organization

Section IV: Methodological Approaches and Cultural Considerations

Chapter 16: Research on Childhood Disability in Jamaica: 1975 to 2005

Molly Thorburn

Introduction

I joined the Department of Pathology of the University of the West Indies (UWI), Jamaica, in 1961 as a trainee pathologist. I had no particular focus initially but quickly developed an interest in paediatric pathology. This soon included cytogenetics which was a new technology developing rapidly at that time especially in the investigation of patients with congenital anomalies and conditions. I contributed to this field during the period 1964 to 1981 with 31 papers and an MD thesis.

The study of genetic and cytogenetic conditions led me into the broader field of the Caribbean and my focus shifted from the laboratory to clinical practice and ultimately into the social aspects. This paper will cover mainly the latter aspects which spanned 30 years. The research can be divided into two aspects, methodological issues and research findings.

Rationale for this Work

In 1970 children with mental retardation and other disabilities comprised the majority of developmental disorders presenting for diagnosis and investigation, but once diagnosed there was no treatment or intervention available and nowhere to refer them for further advice: the parents received a distressing diagnosis but no one could tell them what to do. I began to look at the options and in 1971 I had the opportunity to participate in a very comprehensive seminar in the USA. A group of professionals from a wide range of developing countries were exposed to model programmes for mentally retarded persons including early intervention in the USA. This prompted me to try and develop an early intervention programme in Jamaica. It took 4 years to materialize.

During the 1970s there were political developments in Jamaica that resulted in the facilitation and initiation of early intervention and expansion of special education programmes. These were run by voluntary organisations in the majority but the government began to support the costs. They enabled us to investigate and analyse the priorities for development. This resulted in the initiation of new early intervention and Community Based Rehabilitation (CBR) programmes in most of the island between 1975 and 2000. The difference between early intervention and CBR was the age group covered, the former addressing the 0-6 age group and CBR any age group. The philosophy is the same: that of enabling and empowering families to ensure their children develop to their maximum potential in their own homes and communities. Early intervention alone works where there are other programmes for the older age groups but CBR is ideal for areas that have no disability programmes, which at that time, constituted all Jamaica outside the capital city.

The intent of this paper is to provide an overview and outline the methodologies and scope of intervention used during the period 1975 to 2000. The cultural issues that affected these will be highlighted. The main target group was children with mental retardation and other developmental disabilities. .

Results

These will be reported in two sections, methodologies used and results of intervention.

Part I: Methodologies and Cultural issues in CBR in Jamaica

There were two main groups studieda) detection and assessment of clients and b) survey approaches and situation analyses.

Overview

In order to study the nature and extent of childhood disability, it was necessary to have a methodology that was culturally relevant, accurate, comprehensive and representative of the Jamaican situation and culture. It was clear that the instruments and methods from developed countries such as the USA and UK were culturally inappropriate. An early example of this was a foreign psychologist pronouncing in the 1970s that 30% of Jamaican school age children were mentally retarded because they scored so poorly on standard and culturally inappropriate IQ tests. So we had to reconcile ourselves to using standard instruments and getting biased results, or developing new methodologies more appropriate for developing countries which would take more time and research. We attempted the latter.

Detection and Assessment

Detection

Disability can be and is detected by family members without special methods being used. The normal development of children from soon after birth is of great concern to Jamaican parents and family members. Especially motor milestones are monitored rigorously, though there is much less concern about language and cognitive development. If a child is not sitting up by 4 months of age, the parent or her relatives becomes concerned. As children are seen regularly in child welfare clinics for the first two years of their lives, delays in motor development are detected early. On the other hand cognitive and language delays may not be of concern until well after two years. This means that children may present for basic school at age 3 ½ to 4 years with significant delays in those areas. As there are as yet no standard screening devices to detect delays, children may pass through basic school undetected and move into primary school at a distinct disadvantage.

Since 1981 my colleagues and I have developed and used two main instruments for the detection of childhood disabilities (CDs).

The Ten Questions (TQ) is a screening instrument for detecting CDs in the 2-9 year age group. It was developed for the International Pilot Study on Childhood Disability in 1981 and validated in 3 countries including Jamaica, in the International Epidemiological Study on Childhood Disability (IESCD) between 1987 to 89 (Thorburn et al, 1992a). The test is written in standard English. When we started using it, we thought that it might be more accurate and user friendly if thequestions were in Jamaican patois since the community workers and the majority of the people being screened use that language. To our surprise, the community workers (CWs) using the questionnaire preferred the standard English version, so to our relief the patois version was not used.

We have used the TQin Jamaica since then in two ways:

1. As a screening instrument in the survey of the IESCD
2. As an instrument to be used by CWs to identify the disability in children who were either referred to our programme or who were identified by them in the communities where they were working.

The second one, the Developmental Screening Checklist is a shortened version of the Denver Developmental Screening Test (Frankenburg and Dodds, 1970). The basic difference between this and the TQ is that the TQ uses signs of disability to detect disabilities whereas the DSCL uses delays in development. Because of these differences we have tended to use both tests in any major survey and our clinics.

In 2006, an eleventh question on behaviour was added to the TQ to make it more comprehensive. Since then, we have used it in that form as the Eleven Questions or EQ. This addition has considerably expanded the detection of delays and abnormal results and particularly increases the frequency of detection of behavioural problems which do not surface with the TQ. An advantage of the EQ over the DSCL is that the responses to the questions indicate the type of disability which they do not in the DSCL. On the other hand the latter gives a better estimate of the degree of developmental delay and thus the severity of the disability.

Clinical Assessment

The aim of the clinical assessment of the child with a disability includes the following:

1. To determine whether there is a disability. If so
2. To determine the type and severity of the disability
3. Whether any medical treatment is required
4. What are the areas of developmental delay/problems

5.   To design an intervention programme to meet the needs of #4
6.   To provide counselling and advice to the family to enable them to facilitate the development and management of the child

The following is the protocol for assessment of children with disabilities in our clinics. The procedures are carried out by trained CWs along with a medical assessment by a doctor familiar with the methodology of clinical assessment of the disabled child. The steps and procedures are

1.   The EQ to identify the disability
2.   The DSCL or DDST to estimate the child's developmental level and thus the severity of the disability
3.   The Activities of Daily Living Questionnaire to determine the main ways the disability is negatively affecting the child's development, ie areas of handicap
4.   Medical assessment

From the results of the above, a management plan is drawn up at two levels:

a)   An overall plan to be reviewed over a 2-6 month period. This includesincludes medical and educational procedures and need for appliances, referral or other interventions and further assessments/ referrals if indicated.
b)   A developmental plan to cover day to day intervention activities and to be implemented by the CW assigned to the client. From a cultural standpoint, the fact that this plan is developed and implemented by the CW, as opposed to a professional, makes it more likely that the activities will be more culturally relevant and acceptable than they would be if prescribed by a clinical professional who is not closely acquainted with community issues in the life of the child. So it is more likely to be implemented by the caregiver.

Surveys

Over the years we have been involved in 3 different kinds of survey. These included:

1.   Surveys of clinic case loads, eg analysing the clients attending our clinics over a 5 year period in the early 1970s. This led to us starting the Early Stimulation Project in 1975. Subsequently we analysed other case loads during later years when we started new programmes in other areas. These served to identify the main needs of the local community and also helped us initiate new areas of intervention.
2.   Community surveys to determine the overall nature and extent of the disability problem in different communities. These have consistently shown that mental retardation and developmental disabilities are the most common disabilities in our population. In these surveys we sometimes took a population based approach which identified

asymptomatic persons with disabilities. An example of this would be some children with mild disabilities who would not be recognized unless intelligence testing was done. This type of survey is more comprehensive and detailed but also more costly and time-consuming. It also has important implications since there is an obligation to intervene with the problems that surface, increasing costs and needs for specialized staff.

3. Surveys of defined groups or limited populations sometimes known as situation analyses, eg of clinic populations, institutions or a specific age group. In these the following factors might be investigated;
   a. The specific problem being addressed
   b. Characteristics of the target population
   c. Quantification of the specific problem
   d. Related issues

The following are some of the surveys undertaken during the 20 year period from 1987 to 2007

1. Attitudes towards childhood disability in 3 areas of Jamaica in 1987 (Thorburn, 1998)
2. International Epidemiological Study on Childhood Disability (IESCD)1987to 1989 see below(Thorburn et al, 1992).
3. Situation of disability in the English speaking Caribbean 1983-1997 (Thorburn, 1992).
4. Disabled children in care1992.
5. Survey of disabled children in Bellevue mental hospital 2002.
6. Evaluation of the pre-primary to primary Transitions project in Clarendon 2004 to 2005(Ashby et al, 2005).
7. Developmental and behavioural problems in children entering basic school in 2006. (Thorburn and Windross, 2011).

Part 2: Results of Investigations

This section includes only the Jamaican studies so #2 above is not included. They are reported in chronological order. .

Attitudes towards ChildhoodDisability in 3 Areas in Jamaica (1987)

This was a stratified community survey undertaken to determine existing attitudes and knowledge, prior to commencing a public education programme. The 3 areas each had 300 persons with 5 age and 12 occupational groups. The questions were in 5 main areas, -supernatural beliefs, misconceptions about disability, denial of human rights, competency and willingness to help persons with disabilities and knowledge of disability services.

A minority (18%) held supernatural beliefs with superstitions less prevalent (18%) than the belief that disabled children were "sent by God" (40%). The most negative misconceptions were rejected by an average of 68% though 26% thought that they (CWD) could be a burden at times. Most people were unaware that disabled people could benefit from training in their own homes but 95% felt that programmes should be shared by government and the community. The human rights of persons with disabilities to full participation and equality were only recognized by 50% though the majority (95%) expressed willingness to participate in such programmes. The majority felt that special institutions are best for children with disabilities (Thorburn, 1998).

International Epidemiological Study in Jamaica1987 to 1989

This was a very comprehensive study conducted by the Department of Social and Preventive Medicine of the University of the West Indies (UWI) in collaboration with the Gertrude Sergievsky Centre of New York. The ground breaking range of topics and issues studied can be seen from the list of publications below. (Thorburn et al, 1992 a to d)

Findings

Findings showed that 9.4% of the nearly 1000 2-9 year olds screened were found to have disabilities of which 69% were mild, 19.3% were moderate and 5.6% were severe or profound. Mental retardation accounted for 8.14% of the whole group. However confidence limits were wide indicating that this was only a crude estimate of prevalence. This was due to the relatively low frequency in the population. 30% of these children had twoor more disabilities, of which speech was most frequent.*(Paul et al, 1992).*

Previous Treatment

The responses of the parents regarding previous treatment of their children showed that for all disabilities except epilepsy, only 3-5% had received treatment. Children who had been treeated for epilepsy comprised 87% of the group.

Needs

Needs of disabled children identified were assessed indicating that 62% needed special education, 29.5% neededcommunity based services (CBR), 21% needed referral to a specialist, 21% needed glasses and only 6% required medical treatment (Paul et al, 1992). The majority of these needs could not be met at that time but since then, the expansion of the CBR programme in that area would be expected to meet most of these needs except provision of glasses. This would depend on the parent's ability to buy the glasses.

Disabled Children in Care

This study was done at the request of the Children's Services Department. Approximately 430 children ages 2 to 18 years from residential facilities all over the island were assessed in this study. Nearly 80% were between the ages of 3 and 18 years. These children were not representative of CWDs generally. They were a highly selected group whose homes had broken down leading to their inclusion in care facilities.

The different types of disabilities found were mental retardation in 86%, speech in 70%, physical or motor in 5% and fits, visual and hearing disabilities in 19, 19 and 14% respectively.

At the time of the study there were no remedial or rehabilitative programmes for children in residential care. Some attended special schools where such happened to be available in their locality but there was no integration into regular school programmes. Recommendations for intervention are shown in Table 6.

Table 6: Service Needs of Children in Care

Type of Service	Number needing it	Percent
Specialist referral	114	26
Referral Follow-up	184	42
Integrated schooling	64	15
Specialeducation	193	44
Adaptive aids	52	12
Pre-vocational programme	111	25
Glasses	7	2
Hearing aid	3	1
Home training	290	
Total number of children evaluated	**430**	

I do not know if the above recommendations were implemented.

Survey of Disabled ChildrenIncarcerated in a MentalHospital in Kingston.

The purpose of this study was a needs assessment of the inmates who were housed in the children's ward of the main mental hospital and who were to be transferred to a more suitable children's home where home based training was to be provided. The majority were mentally retarded. They were subsequently relocated and in the new setting, individual intervention programmes based on the assessment were designed.

Evaluation of the Pre-primary to Primary Transitions Project in Clarendon 2004 to 2005

This was a sub-project of a larger study of basic to primary school (ages 3 to 6 years) children in a rural area of southern Jamaica called the Transitions Project conducted by the Ministry of Education. Under-achievement in literacy in Jamaica among school age children has caused national concern for decades and more recently different institutions/organizations have taken a new and closer look at how literacy is taught and learnt. Unfortunately, In spite of enrichment of the curriculum and training of their teachers, basic school children in the Transitions Project in south Clarendon did not perform any better on various measures, than children from non-Transitions schools.

Our component of this investigation sought to identify the factors that might have contributed to this situation. We used the Denver Developmental Screening Test (DDST) to screen the children. The screen positives were then clinically evaluated (Ashby et al, 2005).

Results

16% of children scored suspect on the DDST, 11% of girls and 22% of boys. The history and clinical examination of 80% of the suspect children revealed 7% with moderate mental retardation, the remainder scored between 85 and 106 IQ points. 75% appeared to have emotional problems of various types. Eight children needed medical intervention and 8 appeared to have hearing impairments.

The parent survey was completed by 62% of the parents/caregivers. This indicated a high incidence of poverty, higher proportions of suspect children living with only one or neither of their parents, and a higher incidence of behaviour problems in the suspect children.

It was concluded that the main causes of the failure of the children on the Denver 2 were poverty, associated with cultural factors related to negative child rearing practices and disrupted family structure.

Developmental and Behavioural Problems in Jamaican Children Entering Basic School for the First Time

This study was a more in depth assessment of the children in the previous study and was part of the monitoring and evaluation of the whole Transitions programme. (Thorburn and Windross, 2011)

Screening

The Denver 2 test was used in 2004 to screen 226 children for developmental delays in the 8 basic schools of the project. 16% of this population screened suspect on the second test so that 38 children required evaluation.

The suspect children were boys in 21% and girls in 11% of the sample so there was a significant association with gender. There were no significant associations with age or state of nutrition.

Evaluation

For reasons of time and money only 29 of the 38 suspect children were evaluated. Of this group two were moderately mentally retarded. The rest had cognitive levels of normal -8, low normal 9 and below normal -9. The few health problems identified could have accounted for some of the poor performance, but there were 75% of children with psychological problems including attention deficit disorders and a variety of behaviour problems. Twenty percent of children were living in homes without either parent, another 10% lacked their mothers and 43% lacked their fathers. Only 27% lived in 2 parent families.

The percentage of negative factors in this group of children was much higher than those in a survey done of 160 parents and caregivers of these children in the area.

More detailed analysis of the item scores in the Denver 2 of 40 children indicated that the main items failed were language and the most common failure was in naming of colours. Since normal children can acquire this skill by two years of age, it seems strange that 6 year olds did not know them. It appears to be a common failure in poor Jamaican children.

Conclusions from the Studies

To summarise the above two studies and draw conclusions, we have examined groups of apparently normal children in a rural setting and some of their characteristics and the attitudes towards them. There seems to be a serious problem of under achievement in these poor rural settings. This study confirms many suspicions and previous findings. The results also show that these problems exist already when children commence school and thus originate in the pre-school home environment. The high proportion of children with a single or no parent indicates one of the main underlying cultural problems which are not peculiar to this area.

This cultural pattern is ingrained in the poor component of the Jamaican population and is most likely responsible for the overall high prevalence of poor academic performance and illiteracy in Jamaican children, and which has not shown any real change in recent years. It needs to be addressed by more in depth investigation and intervention into parenting and family practices.

Discussion

The six studies outlined above covered a wide range of problems and perspectives relating to childhood disability in Jamaica in the past 30 years.

Several different cultural influences can be perceived in these studies. These include:

- the influence of language
- supernatural beliefs
- family structure
- poverty

Language

Many children grow up in Jamaica with two languages—English and Jamaican patois. The latter is the first language in poorer homes and they have to acquire Standard English when they start school. Thus they are handicapped in language development and school performance from the beginning. In middle class homes, children are exposed to Standard English from the beginning but also know patois from their household helpers. This English language weakness in the poorest sections of the population is probably one of the main reasons for the high percentage of apparent mental retardation in surveys where Standard English is the main language used in the tests.

Supernatural Beliefs

Supernatural beliefs are common in social groups where parents are poorly educated and don't understand the scientific factors underlying unusual or unexpected features in the problems they encounter in their communities. They seek explanations from their families or close neighbours. Some of these beliefs may be dispelled when they go to school, but where the educational system is weak, the beliefs may persist and get passed on to their children and the cycle continues.

Family Structure

In Jamaica, again most common in the poorest stratum of society, family structure is often weak. This is an inheritance from slavery where family structure was deliberately broken down with the father being kept separate from the rest of the family. Families and family groups more commonly consist of a mother and her children, the latter often having several different fathers, and mayinclude the maternal grandmother. The fathers are frequently itinerant figures or completely absent. This contributes to poverty as well as insecurity. The weakening of the family structure contributes to poor school attendance so the children grow up lacking scientific explanations for unusual occurrences or features thus perpetuating the cycles of superstition.

Poverty

Poverty is the recurring factor in the explanations provided for the peculiarities of mild intellectual disabilities.

Conclusions

This chapter has reviewed the findings of a set of investigations carried out over a 20 year period in a community based rehabilitation programme in rural Jamaica. The main target population was children 0 to 18 years. Some of the main features/ findings from this research included:

1. Need for a relevant methodology in detecting and assessing disability in the community both at the individual and at the community levels.
2. Surveys of different types to identify types and frequencies of different disabilities in different communities. These have included attitudinal andepidemiological studies, assessment of specific groups and their needs, and evaluation of programmes/projects
3. The need to seek, use and evaluate culturally relevant solutions to the problems identified

One feature that needs to be stressed is that all these programmes and methodologies have to be low-cost, otherwise they will not be used in developing countries. In Jamaica, a developing country almost at the top of that scale, many needed programmes have not been implemented or expanded because of cost and what is perceived to be the low priority of CWDs as a target group for intervention. Reports of projects and programmes need to identify and stress their relevance and feasibility in order to be accepted by policy makers as high priority. We still have a long way to go in that respect.

References

Ashby, P, Evans H. and Thorburn, M (2005) Pre-primary to primary Transitions pilot project. Caribbean Journal of Education, vol 25, 156-164

Frankenburg, W., & Dodds, J. (1975). *The Denver Developmental Screening Test – Revised (DDST)*. Denver, CO: University of Colorado Medical Cent

Paul, TJ, Desai,P and Thorburn,MJ (1992) The prevalence of childhood disability and related medical diagnoses in Clarendon, Jamaica. West Ind Med J. 41. 8-11.

Thorburn, MJ (1991) The disabled child in the Caribbean: a situation analysis. West Ind Med. J. 40. 172-179.

Thorburn, M. J. (1992) Training of community workers in a simplified approach to early detection, assessment and intervention. J of Practical Approaches to Developmental Handicap 16. 24-20.

Thorburn, MJ (1993a) Recent Developments in low cost screening and assessment of childhood disabilities in Jamaica. Part 1 Screening W. I. Med J 42, p. 10

Thorburn, MJ (1993b) ditto Part 2 Assessment ibid 42 p46.

Thorburn, M. J.. (1998) Attitudes towards childhood disability in three areas in Jamaica. Asia Pacific Disability Rehabilitation Journal 9: 20-24.

Thorburn, MJ and Paul, TJ (1992) A preliminary report of perinatal risk factors in childhood disability in Clarendon, Jamaica. In Perinatal problems of the islands in relation to the prevention of handicaps. Eds Berchel, Papiernik, de Caunes. Editions INSERM 246-253

Thorburn, M. J. and Windross, M. (2011) Developmental and behavioural problems in Jamaican children entering basic school for the first time International Humanities Review, vol 2, 4-28.

Thorburn, MJ, Desai,P, Paul,TJ, Malcolm,L, Durkin, M, and Davidson,L (1992a) Identification of childhood disability in Jamaica: the Ten Question Screen. Int J of Rehab Research (IJRR) 15. 115-128.

Thorburn, MJ, Desai, P and Paul, TJ. (1992b) Service needs of children with disabilities in Jamaica. Ibid 15, 31-38.

Thorburn, MJ, Desai, P., and Davidson, L. (1992c) Categories, classes and criteria in childhood disabilities. Disability and Rehabilitation 14. 122-132.

Thorburn, MJ, Desai,P, Paul,TJ, Malcolm,L, Durkin, M, and Davidson,L (1992d) Evaluation of the ten question screen. IJRR 15 262-272

Chapter 17: Disability, Research, and Culturally Competent Practice

Mel Stewart

What do we mean by culturally competent research practices and how does this relate to disability? When disability is not the prime area of an investigation in research, how is it captured and reported? This chapter explores associations between disability, research and cultural competence and argues that where disability is not addressed or made more overt in research that internal and external validity could be compromised.

Cohen et al (2011) state that 'internal validity seeks to demonstrate that the explanation of a particular event, issue or set of data which a piece of research provides can actually be sustained by the data'. External validity questions the extent to which this explanation can then be generalised. The concern is, how disability is reflected in research when it is not the main focus of the investigation and how are research methods adapted in order to reflect the true nature of disability in normal populations?

Culturally competent practices are cited across a range of professional practices including education, psychology, sociology and health care. However, within research and more specifically with reference to adjustments for disability in research, reference to it is patchy. Culturally competent practice or cultural competence is said to be a

> ...set of congruent behaviours, attitudes and policies that come together in a system agency or among professionals that enables effective work in cross-cultural situations (Cross et al, 1989 p.28).

Olkin (2002) identifies that despite being the largest minority group, within the multicultural literature, people with disabilities have received less attention than other groups. Limited evidence of the characteristics of disability approaches to managing it and adjustments made for it is given in research literature when the disability is not the main focus. Disability may impact on the research process in a number of ways and omitting it from methods, explanation, evaluation, justification and conclusions drawn could be viewed as negligent (Brown and Boardman, 2011). Additionally, mainstreaming has been identified as a key recommendation in the World Report on Disability (WHO, 2011) where government and stakeholders are called to ensure that persons with disabilities participate equally with others in any activity or service intended for the general public.

Disability within research has been regarded in a number of different and varied ways. The social model of disability identifies physical, social and cultural environments as prime causes for excluding or disadvantaging individuals labelled as disabled (Oliver, 1990) This model has received growing acknowledgment and gained momentum in the 1970's partly aided by the politicisation of disabled people at that time and increasing access of disabled students into higher education through widening participation schemes (Boxall and Beresford, 2012). Influences in the expansion of disability studies amongst academics including those who may be disabled have played their part in promoting this model. User-led disability research has also taken up the baton in promoting it through the use of qualitative research which focuses on emancipatory designs (Beresford 2005). However, whilst this link between disability and environment has been increasingly embraced, there is growing plurality of opinions surrounding this designation (Goodley, 2011). Thomas (2007) would argue that because of the emphasis on the social model, the focus has been taken away from the individual, and that there is still scope to consider restrictions which are directly linked to the individual with impairment. Another view is that disability should include those who have no impairment but suffer discrimination on the grounds of perceived impairment (Beresford et al, 2002). Research appears to take account of these views in varied and sometimes limited ways.

Estimated figures of the number of individuals affected by disability vary but the Department of Works and Pensions estimate the number in Great Britain to be 11.2 million with an unknown number of people remaining unregistered. Across the world, the estimate is considered to be over one billion. Identifying, quantifying and setting classifications of disability continue to pose fundamental problems for those wishing to appropriate numbers and groups to those affected. Categorisation of health status and ability ranges, have come in for much criticism such as within the Olympic and Paralympics Games and especially in the assessment of intellectual and learning abilities (Iacono and Carling-Jenkins, 2012). The International Classification of Functioning Disability and Health (ICF) and in the Convention on the Rights of Persons with Disabilities (CRPD) offer useful guidance including disabilities which are acquired over time, progressive, chronic or aid dependent. Within the UK's Disability Discrimination Act (1995), individuals are considered officially disabled if they have 'a physical or mental impairment which has a substantial and long-term adverse effect on [their] ability to carry out day-to-day activities'. The World Health Organisation identifies disability as 'a complex phenomenon, reflecting an interaction between features of a person's body and features of the society in which he or she lives'. The United Nations Convention on Disability does not employ a fixed definition of disability and sees it as an evolving concept. All of these views highlight some of the complexities associated with understanding disability. Balcazar et al (2010) adds to this in suggesting that we should also recognise the intersection between the multiple identities of disability, race and gender and the extent to which these could impact interpersonal relations between researchers and the subjects and between subjects.

Research Engaging Disabled Communities

The issue of 'hard to reach communities' is commonly cited as one of the problems of conducting research into minority groups and including individuals with a disability. The difficulty is often attributed to the nature of the group rather than the more complex issues of resolving challenges of cultural competence within the research process itself. Bhopal (2012) makes it clear that ethnic minority groups are willing participants in trials once linguistic and trust-related barriers are overcome, though recruitment costs are higher. Similarly, individuals with a disability may be willing participants once reasonable adjustments have been identified and implemented though recruitment costs could also be higher. Whilst researchers might acknowledge the issue of reasonable adjustment through an ethical research code of practice requirements, practical ways for making these adjustments may not be predicted, and researchers' unfamiliarity with barriers in this area may fall short of making appropriate enquiries and explorations regarding how best to engage disabled communities. Ethics committee themselves may lack the expertise to make decisions in some areas of disability (Lai et al, 2006). Eventual outcomes and final reporting of the research could be finalised in thoughts of reasonable adjustments being relegated to statements of 'limitations of the study' or 'ideas for future research'. Therefore, concerns remain regarding conclusions which may be drawn or have been drawn in past investigations and in extrapolations made when levels of disabilities within the recruitment, selection and the research processes remain covert within the research process. Brown and Boardman (2011) concords with this view and make a strong plea for increased openness.

Inclusion and Exclusion Criteria and Disability

Valid and reliable research depends on an in-depth understanding of communities, the characteristics of participants and making explicit relevant measures taken to answer the research question. A lack of openness regarding the reporting of characteristics of subjects with a disability and or populations who are selected and recruited for research when the disability is not regarded as the primary area of the research is of concern. In the recruitment of subjects, self declaration or self-assessment forms are often used to highlight and sift individuals for the investigation. The effectiveness of this process is dependent on ability of potential participants to access the form, the nature of the questions and mode of distribution and in its manner of presentation and other factors. Lack of attention to exploring inclusion of disabled people and other cultural groups could lead to the flawed exclusion of individuals. Potential recruits may find it difficult to ascertain or to decipher whether or not due consideration has been given to active inclusion or exclusion of the disability affecting them. Barriers which could be encountered within a study are often not overtly written and may be assumed not to exist. Accessing publications of forthcoming research, access to buildings and resources are other common areas of concern (Artman and Daniels, 2010). The way in which other challenges such as sexism, racism, ageism interact with disability discrimination in recruitment and selection often go unreported and is cited here as an indication of the complexity surrounding the issues when attempting to make research more inclusive. Indeed, in addressing the issue of 'protected characteristics' of participants in research, it is not always clear the extent to which measures are adopted to address them and to record their impact within the research.

Making Disability Explicit in Research

Even when researchers are health professionals and their work is centred on the individuals who have known disabilities, or they work within a culture where disability is prevalent, the extent and level of their cultural competence (ability to work across different cultural groups) may be unknown. The researcher and research team's experience of working with disability may be left unexplored and unreported within the investigations.

If research is concerned with ontological assumptions (assumptions about the nature of reality) giving rise to epistemological assumptions (ways of researching and enquiring about reality) then implicit within it is an assumption for culturally competent skills. In addition, axiology (values and beliefs) adds to the need to develop increased understanding of what is deemed valuable within and across cultures. Increasing our understanding of the concept of disability and understanding perspectives from which interpretations are made requires inclusion of values of both researcher and the researched. The same may be said to be true for both qualitative and quantitative approaches, yet often in the latter, limited insight of the impact, prevalence and effect of disability amongst the researcher or the participants are ever given when disability is not the focus of the investigation. Researchers with a disability might see it as irrelevant to the study to offer a view on reasonable adjustments within the research. Its impact on the course of the study may not be revealed and so the reader is made none the wiser regarding the interrelationship between disability and how the research evolved. This of course might be deliberate but may have also occurred through unconsidered omission and adds further to the complexity of analyzing the relationship between disability, research and the cultural setting because limited information is available for evaluation. The importance of finding out individuals' conceptual models in terms of their disability, and understanding their social context may be central to understanding how the research evolves and how interactions across the investigation are managed. Brown and Boardman (2011) identify the importance of negotiating 'the disabled body' within the process. The researcher is charged with not only investigating their own stereotypes and prejudices and their impact on the relationships and phases within the study but to also seek out stereotypes and prejudices of other participants and making sense of their interactions within the investigation.

Inclusive Research

Strategies which seek to ensure that disability is appropriately addressed, that reasonable adjustments across the process are not an afterthought, and appropriate reporting regarding disability is included should be a central feature of the research process. However, application and incorporation of strategies may be heavily dependent on the cultural competence of the research team and the development of those skills over the course of the research. It is suggested here that when contemplating 'normal populations' within research, the assumption is made that it is inclusive of disability. The task for the researcher is to consider the extent to which its exclusion might threaten reliability and validity of the study. Based on considerations within the United Nations Convention on the Rights of Persons with Disabilities (UNCRPD) the Convention on the Rights of Persons with Disabilities (CRPD), Equality Act 2010 and the literature, a brief summary of suggestions and guidance is offered below which could assist in making research more inclusive.

Areas for Consideration in Inclusive Research

Accessibility Before, During, and After the Research Study

Ensuring that:

- Publication of the research call for subjects reach diverse communities including a wide spectrum of disabled persons
- Flyers and publication material are available in different formats and is accessible to all
- Due consideration is given to the of use of additional resources and scope of smart phones, speech synthesis, automated voice recognition systems in publicising material and in the call for subjects
- Due consideration is given to access to all buildings
- Websites are structured for easy access and navigation by diverse groups according to the Web Content Accessibility Guidelines (WCAG) and informed from other areas of good practice
- Due consideration is given to the use of assistive technologies (computer software, hardware or tools for accessing information) appropriate to the individual and throughout different phases of the study
- Assumptions regarding individual's ability to read and write is addressed

Study Schedule

- Check appropriateness of instrumentation and their suitability for different groups within a normal population of items e.g. availability of hearing loops etc.
- In terms of reliability, consider whether the same factors will be extracted from the same instrument with different groups of participants i.e. a group with different disabilities?

- Consideraccess to public transportmedication etc. when offering appointments
- Consider use of Skype, computer webcams etc. as additional ways to engage individuals
- Consider lighting, timing of activities to allow for impaired cognition, etc.
- Offer suitable breaks

Interventions

- Consider alternative schedules which are consistent with the research question and without invalidating format of the investigation, for example, improvisation, use of personal support/care workers, making provisions for a guide dog etc.

Service User Support Groups

- Consult and involve relevant groups and stake-holder prior to the study and in setting up the investigations, especially when disability is not the main subject of the investigation

Reporting/Dissemination of ResearchFindings

- Disseminate in formats that can be accessed by disabled communities
- Report measures taken during the study with respect to inclusion, reasonable adjustments etc.
- Make suggestions of further inclusion measures for reaching more diverse groups within the normal population for future research

Applying Equality Impact Assessment

- Conduct an equality impact assessment. This assessment has the potential to identify where individuals might have been unnecessarily excluded, underrepresented and/or disadvantaged.

Addressing the United Nations Convention on the Rights of Persons with Disabilities (UNCRPD)

- Consult the Convention on the Rights of persons with Disabilities (United Nations, 2010) a legally binding treaty which spells out the rights of persons with disabilities where they are invisible in their societies and internationally. It articulates specific social dimension to human rights and emphasises obligation of nations to promote rights and dignities of disabled people.
- Consider respect for person's full and active participation, autonomy, equality of opportunity, accessibility, protection and promotion of rights, developing universally designed services, accessibility including access to information within this Convention as being of equal relevance in research.

Cultural Validity of Research

Different cultural groups respond in systematically different ways which are meaningful to their own culture and context. Hence, in past research where instruments have been shown to be reliable in normal populations where disability was neither contemplated nor acknowledged may now be open to challenge. Additionally, it is often assumed that participants in a research group exhibit the same or similar features of the whole group taken together (Morrison, 2009) and, because of this, findings are often generalized. Great caution should be exercised in doing this, especially when disabilities in its various forms receive limited acknowledgement within the study. Jacobson et al (2005) calls for greater openness in order to enhance reliability and validity and cites the importance of empowering study participants to make decisions concerning the study approach, ensuring mutual respect and trust, appreciating community partners' knowledge, utilisation of expertise and experiences and seeking participant feedback as ways of making research more valid.

The medical model of disability within the healthcare field still remains the dominant approach (Scullion 2010) and so it is one in which disability is often explored. Despite this, it has received limited empirical support (Peterson and Elliott, 2008). Writing from an exploratory research perspective of disability Foley-Nicpon et al (2012) identify that within counselling psychological literature, disability research accounted for an extremely small amount, 1-2.7% of the literature and although there is an increasing move to empirical studies, much of the literature is still based on literature reviews. Approaches which offer scope to make disability more explicit should therefore be considered including pragmatic research and/or multi-methods approaches. Disabled people are also confirming the need for further emancipatory and empowering research designs and strategies (Kitchen, 2002). In the meantime, the literature remains helpful in building additional understanding of the subject and in building a foundation from which future empirical investigations might stem.

Conclusion

In summary, how disability is featured and how adjustments are made for it in research often go unreported unless disability is the focus of the investigation. Limited information is generally given regarding the existence of disability within normal populations. Inclusivity in research is dependent on the cultural competence of researchers and lack of attention to this could threaten reliability and validity of the study. Commitment to shared production between the researched and the researcher arising out emancipatory disability research demonstrates the need for accurate reporting of disability whether or not disability is the main focus of the research. Ensuring that the research environment is enabling and inclusive facilitates individual choices, autonomy and contributions to the process. The warning is that only after assimilating the complexity of individuals' social context, identity, ability and disability should conclusions be drawn from researching them and in making assumptions about human populations.

A Personal Note

My interest lies in seeking to challenge and make evident the scope for further development of cultural competent practices in research and to highlight factors which might question assumptions and perceptions of practices in this area and their potential effect on reliability and validity. It draws upon my status as an individual mwithout a label of disability, my role as a Chartered Physiotherapist, and as a lecturer with experience of exploring culturally competent practices amongst colleagues, students and individuals with disabilities. I accept that individuals with or without disability may challenge some of the assumptions which I make and on the stance I have taken in declaring the issues.

References

Artman, L K and Daniels, J A. Disability and psychotherapy practice: Cultural competence and practical tips. Professional Psychology: Research and Practice, 41(5): 442-448

Balcazar, F E.; Suarez-Balcazar, Y; Taylor-Ritzler, T; et al. (2012) Culture, and disability: Rehabilitation science and practice. Boston, MA, US: Jones and Bartlett Publishers.

Beresford, P., Harrison, C. and Wilson, A. (2002) Mental health, service users and disability: implications for future strategies, Policy& Politics 30(3): 387–96.

Bhopal, R. S (2012) Research agenda for tackling inequalities related to migration and ethnicity in Europe, Journal of Public Health, 34(2): 167-173

Boxall, K. and Beresford, P. (2012) Service user research in social work and disability studies in the United Kingdom. Disability& Society, 1-14

Brown, L. and Boardman, F. K. (2011) Accessing the field: Disability and the research process. Social Science & Medicine, 72 (1): 23-30.

Cohen, L. and Manion, L. (2011) Research Methods in Education. 7th ed. London: Routledge.

Cross, T., Bazron, B. and Dennis, K., et al (1989) Towards a culturally competent system of care: Vol. 1, A monograph on effective services for minority children who are severely emotionally disturbed. Georgetown University (VA): National Technical Assistance Center for Children's Mental Health.

Foley-Nikpon (2012) Disability Research in Counseling Psychology Journals: A 20-Year Content Analysis. *Journal* of *Counseling Psychology, 59(3): 392-398*

Goodley, D. (2011) Disability Studies London: Sage Publications

Farmer, M, and McCleod, F. (2011) Involving disabled people in social research: Guidance by the Office of Disability Issues. HM Office for Disability issues.

Iacono, T. and Carling-Jenkins, R. (2012) The human rights context for ethical requirements for involving people with intellectual disability in medical research. Journal of Intellectual Disability Research56 (11): 1122.

Kitchen, R. (2000) The Researcher Opinions on Research: disabled people and disability research. Disability and Society, 15 (1): 25-47.

Lai, R., Elliott, D. and Oullette-Kuntz, H. (2006) Attitudes of research committees towards individuals with intellectual disabilities: the need for more research. Journal of Policy and Practice in Intellectual Disabilities 3, 114–18.

Morrison, K. R. (2009) Causation in Educational Research. London: Routledge

Olkin, R. (2012) Could you hold the door for me? Including disability in diversity. Cultural Diversity and Ethnic Minority Psychology, 8(2): 130-137

Oliver M. (1990)The politics of disablement. Basingstoke, Macmillan and St Martin's Press.

Oliver, M. (1983) Social Work with Disabled People. Basingstoke McMillans

Thomas, C. (*2007*) Sociologies of *Disability* and Illness. Contested Ideas in *Disability* Studies and Medical Sociology. Basingstoke: Palgrave Macmillan.

Scullion, P. A. (2010). Models of disability: Their influence in nursing and potential role in challenging discrimination. Journal of Advanced Nursing, 66, 697–707

United Nations (2010) Convention on the Rights of Persons with Disabilities http://www.un.org/disabilities/default.asp?id=259 accessed 3/5/13

World Health Organisation (2011) World Report on Disability. http://whqlibdoc.who.int/publications/2011/9789240685215_eng.pdf accessed 10/5/13

Chapter 18: Disability and Culture: The Way Forward

Patricia Smith

As we look to the future, it is clear that several issues need to be addressed for those living with disability in different cultures. There are underlying inequalities in how people with disability are treated and catered for in society. Chapter 2 has outlined these inequalities giving its readers a clear indication and explanation of the causative factors and possible solutions. The disparity between the needs of the disabled and provisions for the disabled, calls for a greater emphasis being made to balance the playing field between the disabled and the able-bodied. This can be achieved by creating models of practice which puts people living with disability at the centre of health care, thereby removing barriers to integration and full participation in society (WHO, 2011).

These barriers are not only in daily activities of living and socio-economic advances, but also in sport, an area of life that encourages participation, and is culturally significant (Chapter, 3). Sport not only improves health and well-being but also encourages a sense of achievement and excellence, for all people including those living with disabilities. Hence society's responsibility to provide positive representation of the disabled in the media is an important element in breaking down marginalization of the disabled and developing a culture of acceptance and unity for all people including those living with disabilities.

Chapter 4 looked at how mental health as a disabling factor some has stigmatized, marginalized, disenfranchised many people. Mental health is important to man's well being in life and evidence of how good mental health impact on a person's life is in seen in the programmes of community based projects in countries such as Sri Lanka. There is a need to take this model further, to develop similar yet culturally appropriate models in other regions of the world.

In other developing countries what is very prominent is the effects of post-colonialism on a culture. Post-colonialism has inherent within it a dominant imperial culture which imposed on an existing culture often to the detriment of the subjugated culture (chapter 5). Disability in the context of post-coloniality therefore brings its own unique set of issues as the framework of post-colonialism or neo-colonialism colours how people in developing countries view their health and disabilities. These issues have been evidenced in people living with disability in post-colonial Jamaica where they face experience of issues such as resistance, suppression and loss of cultural identity, poverty, crime, breakdown in family structure, war and conflict. People at all levels in such a society therefore need to find ways through their own creative genius and spiritual cultivation to re-build their reality of independence, which allows those living with disability to realize their full potential.

Chapters 6 and 10 have provided, through a discourse on cultural competence, a means for helping professional gain an understanding of how they can help those living with disability realize their fullest potential. Cultural competence provides a framework for how professional should approach disability in different cultural contexts. Like any skill, cultural competence needs to be taught and it is suggested that professional going out to work in cultures other than their own, should examine how they can improve their levels of competence in order to achieve the best outcomes for their patients.

As we go across cultures as seen in the second section of this book it is noted that a common theme that permeates throughout the chapters is the need for those living with disability *to be acknowledged*. It is not just about acknowledging the disability but acknowledging the fact that those living with disability are beings with unlimited potential to achieve their goals in life as anyone else as long as there is equity and fairness in all aspects of daily living. This book also highlights that for those living with disability the social and family network play an integral part of their lives and is evident in the cultural imperatives of each society. There are cultural imperatives that dictate how families work together, how they create relationships, how they engage with disability.

In the case of disability, the worth, value and importance of that child, woman, man to the family and the community will influence how those living with disability remain an integral part of family, community and social life. Whichever part of the world that person lives, there is a set of values and norms that allows them to be seen and valued and given pre-eminence in society, whether it is through the education system, the health systems, though advocacy groups for governments involvement and policy development, voluntary groups, parents groups, to name a view. They all have in common the desire to *create possibilities and potentials* for those disenfranchised by society because of a disability. The way forward therefore is for professionals along with community workers, family members, special interest organizations, NGOs and government bodies to continue keeping this important issue on the agenda in the next decade and beyond and to make available the resources to bring these potentials into realization.

However, the underlying theme from all this is about understanding self, that infinite potential to realize one's goals in life, to be successful, to achieve, to live and the *enjoyment of living*! The spirit of community and community capacity building as evidenced in the 3D Community Based Rehabilitation Project in Jamaica, (Chapter 7), the Women's Project of Sri Lanka (Chapters 4) and the narrative on one woman being able to transform her own reality of living with multiple sclerosis towards a level of independence through fortitude (Chapter 8) are but examples of this. In addition with the help of professionals in motivating and encouraging those with disabilities to engage in exercises (Chapter 9), self-blaming and punishment beliefs around disability need not become the focus of those living with disability. Instead the focus becomes achieving one's goal and living a life of health and well being.

The debate around culture and disability is further highlighted when we look at the almost diametrically opposed cultural views on disability from an Eastern and Western perspective, (Chapter 13). The notion of disability can be framed within any of these perspectives through thoughts such as, "I am disabled because I have done wrong" or "I am disabled therefore you owe me". Whatever the thinking, the bottom line is those living with disability *need and want to be heard*. What able-bodied people in society hears may be a different matter. Do those in society hear the cry of those living with disability, or do they hear their own discomforts, biases, assumptions and inabilities about disability? As we forge our way forward in the years to come and as we try to understand the relationship between culture and disability, some of these challenges may need to be addressed through appropriate and meaningful lines of communication. Whether these communication gateways are implemented through government policy, education of healthcare professionals on disability, support from non-governmental organizations, the voice of advocates on disability rights advocates advocates that the aim is to keep the needs of those living with disability on the agenda.

The life long journey to cultural proficiency as described in chapter 10 gives us a key to some of these questions. For example professionals in rehabilitation need to have a working knowledge of socio-cultural domains, an appreciation of material conditions in which culture exists, such as the physical environment both in terms of terrain, political-economic (poverty, affluence, war and crisis), infrastructure and economics (buildings, transport, housing) the social and family relationships, and aspects of culture such as values and beliefs and spirituality. Taboos around disability, e.g. in a post-apartheid South Africa is rift with poverty and harshness in rural communities and one which sees traditional healers as a recognized part of the health care system epitomizes what can be seen as a forging of differing western and traditional cultural values and beliefs within a country in order to meet the needs of its' population. Similarly in other countries such as India the statistics have shown that poverty is one of the causes of disability (chapter 14) and disability is a main cause of poverty. In moving forward governments have to look at the socio-economic factor around disability and the resources that are needed to assist the disabled. In other societies divided along religious lines such as in the Palestinian territories, disability is embedded in a patriarchal framework influenced by Islamic and minor Christina religion (Chapter 15). They too see disability as a shame on the family because of the importance of physical beauty in social institutions such as marriage.

As we look at these many examples of the thinking around disability in different culture, fundamental to the issues discussed is *self-knowledge*. Knowledge of self is a dominant cultural imperative in any society and implicit within it are ideas of universality. How these ideas are expressed in different cultures is another matter and is worth further investigation in the future.

Needless to say, it has been pointed out in previous chapters that cultural competency will become a priority in educational institutions that train professionals in the field (Chapter 10) as there will be challenges with placing newly qualified graduates in demanding health care environments.

Last but not least, the way forward calls for more research in the area of disability and culture. Not only is research needed around disability and culture, but research needs to be done around providing the methodological approaches that can address disability and culture in a rigorous, scientific manner. This will provide the evidence needed to inform health care professionals in their decision making process when changing practice. Chapters 16 and 17 discuss this and hopefully leave the reader with the understanding that the culture of research must be in line with the culture of the times. This will enhance the appropriateness and relevance of findings to the cultures being researched. It will stand up to scrutiny and provide a platform for debate and discussion. More needs to be done on this as we move forward into the future.

Disability can be seen as a universal concept as people are people wherever they live in the world, but culture determines *how* disability is perceived and therefore addressed in different societies. All that has been discussed in this book calls for professionals, policymakers, managers, governments, voluntary organizations, practitioners, researchers, students, service users and families alike to give serious consideration to their roles in providing a future where those living with disability can enjoy a full and rewarding life in their respective countries and do so in a culturally appropriate manner that addresses and meets their needs.

Reference

WHO (2011) World Report on disability. World Health Organization& World Bank.

Index

A

Access, 118, 126
Accessibility, 91, 115, 119, 170
Accident, 131
Acupuncture, xii, 132, 134, 135
Age, 133
AIDS, 106, 122, 126, 127
Analysis, 27, 31, 173
Apartheid, 27
Assessment, 104, 156, 157, 165, 171
Attitudes, x, 45, 61, 107, 110, 128, 159, 165, 174

B

Barriers, 15, 16, 17, 84, 168
Beliefs, 58, 60, 164
Benhabib, 2, 48, 50, 51, 53, 58, 59, 72, 76, 77
Bill of Rights, 124
Biological, 45
Blindness, 140, 141
Blood, 130
British Empire, 48
Buddha, 128
Buddhism, 106, 128

C

Caribbean, 47, 49, 52, 60, 78, 116, 155, 159, 165
Census, 121, 122, 127, 138, 139, 140, 141, 142, 144, 145, 147
Cerebral palsy, 145
Childhood, x, 17, 61, 155, 157, 159
Children, xv, 8, 36, 42, 43, 45, 46, 54, 61, 69, 74, 106, 108, 109, 125, 160, 161, 162, 173
China, x, xii, 128, 129, 131, 132

Chinese, x, xii, 10, 53, 106, 128, 129, 130, 131, 132, 135
Chinese Herbal Medicine, xii
Chinese massage, 129, 131
Christian, 58, 87, 94, 106, 148, 152
Christianity, 87, 148
Clinicians, 64
Commonwealth, 31, 49
Communication, 25, 27, 28, 29, 30, 59, 93, 117
Communitarian, 3, 77, 78
Communities, 4, 8, 14, 15, 17, 168
Community, 4, ix, 2, 3, 33, 37, 39, 40, 44, 45, 47, 48, 56, 59, 60, 71, 73, 76, 77, 78, 114, 151, 158, 176
Community Based Rehabilitation, ix, 33, 40, 44, 47, 48, 60, 71, 76, 78, 176
Concrete Other, 75
Conflict, 3, 37, 150
Confucianism, 128
Consciousness, 3
Coping, 30, 59
Crisis Zone, x, 148, 150
Cross Cultural Adaptability Inventory (CCAI), 104
Cross-cultural, 23, 108, 119, 152
Cultural, ix, x, 17, 26, 28, 29, 33, 44, 45, 49, 50, 53, 54, 59, 60, 62, 63, 65, 66, 68, 69, 71, 78, 85, 87, 89, 90, 98, 99, 100, 101, 102, 103, 104, 105, 107, 108, 109, 110, 154, 156, 172, 173, 174, 176
Cultural blindness, 66
Cultural Competence, ix, x, 62, 63, 65, 66, 68, 69, 78, 98, 99, 100, 101, 103, 104, 105, 107, 108, 109, 173, 176
Cultural Competence Health Practitioner Assessment (CCHPA), 104, 108

www.ingramcontent.com/pod-product-compliance
Lightning Source LLC
Chambersburg PA
CBHW032137020426
42334CB00016B/1194